Compassionate Touch

Ms. Nelson has outlined, in easily readable fashion and with attention to practical detail, how to become fully engaged with the elderly and the ill. Essential reading for all caregivers!

Dr. George Fong
Director, Internal Medicine Residency Program
Kaiser Permanente Hospital, Martinez, Calif.

The hands-on health care guidance in this book goes straight to the heart! The world would be a better place if more people read and practiced the gift of Compassionate Touch.

Michael Reed Gach
author of *Arthritis Relief at Your Fingertips*

Here are tools for revolutionizing geriatric care and utterly transforming the personal experience of aging in America.

Deane Juhan
author of *Job'sBody: A Handbok for Bodywork*

The author's experience and compassion fill her book with practical information and unique insight for enriching the client-practitioner relationship. This book is invaluable to all in the health care field.

Dr. Daniel Karan & Dr. Sallie MacNeill
MacNeill & Karan Chiropractic, Oakland, Calif.

The evidence of intuition is through the tasks on which it depends. Dawn conveys tools of the task that has shaped her genuine connection to the source.

Helen Palmer
author of *The Enneagram: Understanding Yourself and the Others in Your Life*

This book presents to me a fresh and new way of appreciating Buddhist icons, particularly the open, extended hands of the Buddhas which traditionally have symbolized sharing, intrinsic to the Buddhas' wisdom and compassion. Dawn Nelson has extended the scope of this sharing in her personal experiences of working with the aged and the infirm.

Dr. Kenneth K. Tanaka
Associate Professor, Institute of Buddhist Studies, Berkeley, Calif.
author of *The Dawn of Pure Land Chinese Buddhist Doctrine*

Offers all caregivers new ways to deepen and communicate their caring.

Dr. Dale G. Larsen
Santa Clara University, Santa Clara, Calif.

Compassionate Touch

Compassionate Touch

Hands-On Caregiving
for the Elderly, the Ill and the Dying

Dawn Nelson, M.F.A.,C.M.T.

FOREWORD BY DEANE JUHAN

Station Hill Press

Published by Station Hill Press, Inc., Barrytown, New York, 12507.
Text and cover design by Susan Quasha, assisted by Vicki Hickman.

All photographs, copyrighted in the names of the photographers, are used here by permission.

Distributed by the Talman Company, 131 Spring Street, Suite 201E-N, New York, New York 10012.

Library of Congress Cataloging-in-Publication Data

Nelson, Dawn, 1943-
   Compassionate touch : hands-on caregiving for the elderly, the ill, and the dying / Dawn
   Nelson.
        p. cm.
   Includes bibliographical references and index.
   ISBN 0-88268-149-4 : $17.95
   1. Touch—Therapeutic use. 2. Massage—Therapeutic use. 3. Aged—Care. 4. Terminal care.
   I. Title.
   RZ999.N38 1994
   615.8'22—dc20   93-48423
                                                          CIP

Manufactured in the United States of America.

for my teachers, in their many forms

Contents

Foreword

During an era when Americans over 60 years old are rapidly becoming the largest single sector in our population, practical, effective, and compassionate approaches to their special health care problems can only become increasingly imperative. Dawn Nelson's work brings to these individuals one of the most promising palliatives available: competent, caring, nurturing—and therapeutic —human contact.

There is no "cure" for the aging and dying processes; and, indeed, most of the measures currently applied to them are both ruinously expensive and ultimately dehumanizing, adding days to lives but not quality to days. Touching, listening, comforting, and relieving isolation, chronic pains, stresses, and fears are frequently the most significant gifts that can be given to any of us as we confront our inevitable deterioration and mortality.

Both the novice and the trained professional will find a wealth of instruction for safely and effectively addressing the unique physical and emotional needs and frailties of the elderly. Here are the tools for revolutionizing geriatric care and utterly transforming the personal experience of aging in America.

Deane Juhan
author of *Job's Body*

Acknowledgements

My deepest gratitude and respect go to those individuals who allow me to know them through my practice of Compassionate Touch. Some are close to leaving their bodies at the time we meet and invite me to share in those sacred, precious moments of their lives. Others become unique and special friends as we work together over time.

My oldest daughter, Brianna, continually instructs and inspires me in the compassionate, skillful way she relates to the elderly and the ill in her care. She has helped me tremendously in creating Compassionate Touch as an outreach program, and I am truly grateful for her ongoing encouragement, support, and advice.

I am grateful to those individuals who allowed photographs to be taken during our sessions together—Adelle, Anna, Bill, Bob, Catherine, Eleanor, Everett, Frances, Gayle, Harry, Josephine, Monty, Robert, and William—and to those who photographed them—Barry, Bonnie, Brock, George and Hunter. I also thank Michael Pedersen for taking and sharing photos of his wife during her illness and last few weeks of life.

I am indebted to Skanda, who taught me what true compassion is and who continues to educate, encourage, and enlighten me, in evolving as an individual. I am grateful to Stephen Levine who has inspired me as well as countless others, to meet our fears with mercy, to awaken before we die, and to die into life.

A special thank you to Susan McAdam for welcoming me as a hospice volunteer and for putting me to work. Thanks, also, to Claire Wasser for meticulous proofreading, and to Pat Curtain for his computer wisdom and generosity. I thank Ron Valle for his pioneering vision in creating a unique academic training program to facilitate Awakening to Life and Death.

I am particularly grateful to my husband Barry, for his daily support, friendship, and love, for his commitment to living life as a spiritual practice, for enriching my journey in countless ways. I thank my son Michael for his gentle wisdom and for calling out the best in me. I thank sweet Meghan—for her bright and shining presence, and for bringing me into the sacred fire of her unending love.

Preface

Much has been made of the fact that physical, human contact is crucial during the early stages of life. Research done on institutionalized infants has proven that those who are deprived of caring touch fail to thrive and soon become emaciated. I believe that those in later life stages who are similarly deprived of tender and nurturing physical contact experience a diminishing quality of life, a lessening of their desire to relate to others, and a weakening of what may already be a fragile relationship with reality.

Being touched in a way that is healing, nourishing, relaxing, and pleasurable is an experience largely denied the ill and the aged in our society. No longer sexually active, the only kind of physical contact many such people receive is in the form of medical attention.

I developed Compassionate Touch as a form of hands-on, palliative therapy and comfort care specifically for individuals who are less active due to aging and/or illness. I visit individuals in retirement communities, nursing homes, convalescent and extended care facilities, hospital and medical centers, and private homes. Some of the people I see are recovering from surgical or other invasive medical procedures and/or various illnesses. Some are disabled, some chronically or acutely ill, some are confronting life-threatening diseases such as cancer or AIDS, and some are actively dying. I also work with individuals who are simply nearing the end of their life's journey and are growing naturally weaker. Some of the individuals I see are no longer able to communicate verbally. Others derive pleasure from our social interaction, enjoy talking, and are grateful for an active listener. A large percentage of the people I work with are in pain, whether it be physical, emotional, mental, or spiritual. Their discomfort is often alleviated by the intimate contact we share through Compassionate Touch.

This book is offered as a resource for any individual who finds her or himself, by conscious choice or through life experience, in an ongoing relationship with someone who is seriously ill, aging, and/or entering a final stage of life. The book is intended as a help for health care professionals, volunteer caregivers, family members, and anyone else who works in close contact with the ill and/or the elderly. It is also meant to be a supportive guide for massage therapists and bodyworkers who want to expand or develop their skills in the area of geriatric massage and/or working with the seriously ill. The later chapters, in particular, are instructional in nature for those who wish to practice this particular kind of attentive touch and care.

Touch is essential to the quality of our existence. It gives comfort, warmth, pleasure, renewed vitality, and assurance that we are not alone. It is my hope that this book will expand the reader's awareness of the nurturing and healing potential of hands-on contact and that it will serve both as an encouragement and as a reminder of the myriad ways that we can all benefit from compassionate care in the form of touch.

My work is challenging, rewarding, and enlightening. I learn a great deal from the people I touch—about life, about process, about surrender, about healing, about grace, about being. I have learned that people can live until they die, that every step of our journey truly is an opportunity for awakening, and that death is not necessarily the end of anything.

Dawn Nelson
January 1992
Walnut Creek, California

❧ 1 ❧

Introduction

I believe that at every level of society — familial, tribal, national and international — the key to a happier and more successful world is the growth of compassion. We do not need to become religious, nor do we need to believe in an ideology. All that is necessary is for each of us to develop our good human qualities.

The Dalai Lama of Tibet

Compassionate Touch, as outlined in this book, is a gentle, sensitive, and non-intrusive program of massage, attentive touch, and supportive comfort care created specifically for those individuals who are temporarily or permanently less active. This includes people who are entering later life stages through a natural aging process as well as those who are acutely or chronically ill, disabled, or injured. It also includes individuals of any age who are actively beginning the mysterious life transition that we call death.

Compassionate Touch comprises, yet is not limited to, certain therapeutic massage techniques. It is a hands-on practice in the form of physical contact, yet it touches more than the body. It reaches beyond that which can be seen. Compassionate Touch emanates not from the hands but from the heart. In Compassionate Touch, massage and attentive touch techniques are combined with other nonverbal and verbal skills such as active listening, reflective communication, intuitive feedback, guided relaxation, and breathing awareness exercises.

Having compassion for another implies experiencing a feeling of unconditional regard for that other; it also implies a genuine, sincere interest in that person's well-being. The compassionate heart shares in, and is affected by, the suffering of another. Compassion supports an ability to offer appropriate aid or assistance when it is needed. The compassionate individual is able to put aside his or her own concerns for a time in order to give attention to someone else. Some say compassion is love in action.

Compassionate Touch is hands-on contact that is given with particular care and attention, not just to the physical condition of the recipient but to that individual's psycho-social, emotional, and spiritual needs as well. Compassionate

Touch may be administered to individuals who are experiencing intense physical discomfort and mental anxiety, along with psychological and emotional trauma. Pain increases fear and anxiety. Feelings of anger, helplessness, isolation, and frustration are likely to surface when expectations are unmet or when events occur that push the ego/mind beyond its current boundaries of thought. Compassionate Touch is one way of providing contact, reassurance, relief, and comfort for those who may be feeling frightened, depressed, out of control, abandoned, overwhelmed, confused, or in despair.

In the aged, in particular, the course, as well as the duration, of many minor diseases can be greatly influenced by the quality of tactile support and care the individual receives. In administering Compassionate Touch, the goal is not only to promote relaxation, reduce stress, and provide aid in the relief of pain, but to help nurture, nourish, support, and comfort. Compassionate Touch is healing touch—not healing in the sense of reversing the aging process or of taking away a disease or a disability, but healing in the broader sense of acceptance that allows awareness to expand beyond physical or mental discomfort to a larger reality of wholeness and well-being.

Compassionate Touch can be administered by anyone who feels inspired to reach out toward a fellow human being in need. Indeed, the impulse to share our energy through touch often arises spontaneously and intuitively when our hearts open to those around us who are yearning for contact and in need of acknowledgement. Anyone can cultivate the natural compassion of the heart. Specific skills can then be learned, or inherent abilities expanded, in order to practice the powerful and compassionate art of loving and healing through touch.

The Compassionate Touch practitioner must constantly create, adapt, and re-create appropriate techniques in administering to the unique needs of the aging and/or the seriously ill individual depending on the situation, condition, or state that person may be in at any given moment. There can be no rigid rules, there are no easily delineated steps to follow in administering Compassionate Touch. Compassionate Touch is a way of relating *to* others rather than a prescribed set of techniques to be practiced *on* others. It is a spontaneous experience of relationship that must unfold moment to moment.

The key to both individual inner peace and planetary balance, on all levels, may well be the growth of compassion. The Dalai Lama of Tibet, winner of the Nobel Peace Prize and a man who has touched people's hearts around the world by his simple and profound message of universal responsibility and great compassion, has said that he has only one real practice: he makes an effort to treat each person he meets as an old friend. This gives him a genuine feeling of happiness. It is through such a practice that true compassion and loving-kindness flow.

The experience of compassion may lead to actively supporting or assisting another in some way, doing something for him or her, as in the case of administering attentive touch, or it may mean just being consciously present with that person. It may mean listening and understanding to the best of one's ability, what another person needs to communicate about himself or about her experience. It may mean letting go of preconceived ideas, opinions, expectations, and agendas in order to remain open and attentive to the individual who is experiencing pain and anguish or to one who is simply feeling alone or isolated. Compassion may mean nothing more than accepting the reality of a situation and being willing to remain consciously present, for even a few moments, in that reality with another human being.

In truth, compassion is not something we *have for* another being. It is rather an experience *of* being. Ultimately, we cannot feel unconditional regard, love, or compassion for another, we can only *be* unconditional love.

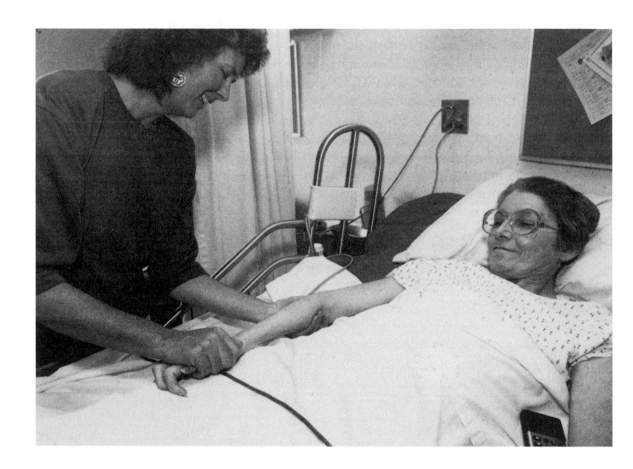

❦ 2 ❦

Benefits and Effects of Compassionate Touch

It is well known in professional circles that young nursing students tend to avoid touching elderly patients, and especially the acutely ill . . . touching as a therapeutic event is not as simple as a mechanical procedure or a drug, because it is, above all, an act of communication . . . The use of touch and physical closeness may be the most important way to communicate to acutely ill persons that they are important as human beings.

Ashley Montague

With the great variety of advanced medical techniques and pain relieving drugs available in our modern world, we tend to forget that the simple, *care*-full touch of the human hand is one of the most ancient and effective means for relieving discomfort in the body, reducing stress, and inducing a state of relaxation. Attentive touch, administered consciously and lovingly, can also facilitate emotional release, calm the mind, lift the spirit, and help restore a sense of worth and balance to a troubled, anxious soul. Compassionate Touch can be of enormous benefit to those whom it serves in any number of physical, emotional, psychological, social, and even spiritual ways.

Compassionate Touch often fulfills several different needs simultaneously. Massage has been proven useful as a primary or adjunct therapy for any condition that includes a stress component in people of all ages. A reduction in bodily tension promotes an overall relaxation response, which, in turn, can produce benefits such as greater ease in breathing, greater mobility, and an increase in appetite. As tension and stress are relieved, minor physical ailments often disappear.

During a Compassionate Touch session, the general level of nervous tension is almost always reduced. This can decrease muscle contraction, increase circulation, and produce a lower heart rate and blood pressure. These changes contribute to a lessening of anxiety and promote relaxation, which can effectively soothe the body, quiet the mind, and strengthen the spirit. In other words, the relaxation response causes a chain reaction of positive benefits within the body/mind.

Improvements in Bodily Functions

In general, therapeutic massage techniques serve to improve circulation in the body, alleviate discomfort from tight muscles and joints that may be swollen and stiff from disuse, and promote an overall relaxation response in the body. In addition, massage and attentive touch can be used as a therapeutic aid for treating specific conditions or problems.

Insomnia can be caused from any number of physical and emotional distresses as well as from environmental conditions. A person's inability to sleep well can become an additional source of stress for that individual as well as for his or her caregivers. Compassionate Touch has a tranquilizing effect on many people. As the body relaxes and tensions ease, a person may be able to breathe more easily and more deeply. Greater ease in breathing can facilitate more tranquil and restful sleep. It is not uncommon for a client to doze off during a Compassionate Touch session; in fact, massage therapy has been known to replace the need for sleep-inducing medications.

There are many reasons for loss of appetite in those who are aged and/or ill. Drug and chemotherapy treatments, constipation, nausea and vomiting, pain, weakness and fatigue, mouth problems, and liver and pancreatic disorders can all affect the appetite. Certainly anxiety and depression often affect one's desire to eat. A reduction in stress and better circulation in the body can promote better digestion as well as increase a natural desire for food and drink.

Constipation is a common problem among the aging and those suffering from various diseases. This is most often due to inactivity, lower fluid intake, and/or the effect of medications. It is a problem that can be extremely irritating, frustrating, and uncomfortable. Constipation is usually treated through diet and/or mild laxatives. Gentle abdominal massage can be helpful in stimulating bowel activity. Reducing a person's general stress level and overall state of anxiety and increasing circulation in the body can also help ease elimination problems.

Long-term immobility and/or illness inevitably leads to poor circulation, which can in turn create other symptoms such as inertia, shortness of breath, loss of appetite, mental confusion, and even depression. Therapeutic massage stimulates the nervous system and increases the oxygen-carrying capacity of the blood throughout the body. Patients often experience greater ease in breathing and are able to rest or sleep more easily after a Compassionate Touch session. They may experience increased mental clarity and often feel less despondent and more "alive."

The news media recently reported that new research with a group of individuals diagnosed as HIV positive is showing that massage and touch therapy may boost the immune system. This news has far-reaching implications in the search for ways to ward off opportunistic infections in those with compromised immune systems who are working to maintain physical health and balance.

Since injured tissues must have oxygen to rebuild themselves, massage also aids in the rehabilitation and upkeep of the tissues. Patients are encouraged to get up and walk as soon as possible after surgical procedures because any form of movement will increase circulation, and increased circulation speeds healing and recovery. Massage techniques that help promote better circulation in the body and prevent the buildup of harmful toxins also contribute to this healing process.

Help in Prevention of Skin Problems

Loss of skin elasticity and dryness are natural effects of aging. Dehydration, immobility, some medications, and a generally rundown condition also contribute to skin degeneration. Moisturizing the skin frequently becomes more important as the aging process continues, as does the need for tactile stimulation.

One of the most persistent problems of confinement and decreased mobility is susceptibility to bedsores. Bedsores occur when an area of skin loses its blood supply for an extended period of time. When a prominent part of the body, such as the spine, lies against a surface like a mattress, nutrients and oxygen are prevented from reaching the skin cells of that particular area. Sitting or lying in the same position for long periods of time puts a great deal of constant pressure on the skin. Other parts of the body especially prone to bedsores include the tailbone, shoulders, elbows, buttocks, heels, and ankles. The skin in those areas can become red and painful fairly quickly, and the skin cells may eventually die if there is no relief from the pressure.

One of the main reasons that nurses and other caregivers are instructed to turn patients or to encourage them to shift their body positions every few hours is to ward off skin ulcerations. Massaging areas of the body that have been most recently under pressure and thus stimulating circulation to those points will also help prevent bedsores. Massaging a cream into red areas as soon as they appear can help keep this problem under control.

Objects pressed against the skin over a long period of time, such as a watch or even a tube connection, can also cause redness and irritation. This discomfort can be easily alleviated by shifting the position of the object and renewing circulation in that area.

Itching is another condition that can occur as a result of skin breakdown, medication, dehydration, allergic reactions, and any number of other causes. Moisturizing and massaging the skin may help alleviate this annoying symptom. If the condition persists, a medicated or topical cream may be needed. Do not, of course, massage over an itching or weeping rash that could be contagious or which you might spread to other parts of the body. If you are in doubt about whether a skin condition is contagious, find out before touching or massaging directly on that place.

Psoriasis is one inflammatory skin disease that can look quite alarming in its acute state. It is characterized by reddish patches and white scales and can cause itching. Psoriasis, however, is not contagious and gentle massage over such a condition can be extremely soothing to the sufferer.

It is good for the skin to be kept clean and dry. Sweating is a fairly common problem for the ill. It can occur for no apparent reason or it may be caused by anxiety, reaction to medication, sudden changes in body metabolism, or fever. A little powder sprinkled and lightly massaged into the skin in areas of the body susceptible to sweat, such as under arms or large breasts, can help with this problem.

Pain Relief

Most seriously or chronically ill patients experience some degree of physical discomfort and pain during the course of their disease and treatment. The pain can be severe, chronic, and debilitating. Anxiety and depression can intensify the perception of pain. Drug therapy is one of the major modalities used in managing pain, but drug therapy alone is seldom very effective, especially in cases where there is bone or nerve involvement. In more enlightened medical communities, massage is now considered an adjunctive measure for comfort control in the palliative treatment of medical conditions diagnosed as "terminal." More and more hospice organizations are making an effort to include massage therapy in the services they offer. Some doctors have also begun to recognize that massage can hasten a patient's overall recovery period from acute illness and lessen the pain caused by muscular tension related to the stress of traumatic injury and/or surgery.

According to a recent article in the *Boston Globe* by Richard A. Knox, a federal panel assigned by the U.S. government to study ways to improve medical care and lower costs urged greater use of drug alternatives such as massage and relaxation techniques in their guidelines. Hopefully, such studies will encourage more health care professionals to prescribe therapeutic massage for help in pain management, rather than relying on potent and expensive drugs, which often have serious side effects that must then be treated with more drugs!

Massage is also helpful in reducing painful tension and muscle spasms that are the result of injury or of years of stored up and repressed emotions. The sedative effects of massage cause a reflex reaction of the nerves that decreases muscle tension. This sedative effect on the nerves may also account for the decrease in pain impulses carried by the nerves to the brain.

Nurses and other caregivers have observed that patients' need for pain medication is often reduced after a Compassionate Touch session. The reduction in pain after attentive touch and massage may occur for a number of different reasons. It may be because the stimulation has improved circulation in a particular area, allowing energy to flow more freely and thus relieve some of the discomfort. It may be that the tender loving care the patient has experienced through his contact with another has allowed him to relax and soften to the point of becoming more accepting of his pain. In general, as the person relaxes that individual often finds his or her condition less stressful and more tolerable.

Stress Reduction and Relaxation

Stress is thought to be a major factor in causing hypertension, coronary heart disease, migraine headaches, ulcers, and asthmatic conditions. Stress is associated with gastrointestinal disorders such as colitis and gastritis, is found to be a factor in many skin diseases, and aggravates almost any chronic health condition. Some of the excess hormones released by the adrenal glands during repeated stress responses can lower the body's immunity making one more susceptible to bacterial infections and viruses such as flu.

For the aged residents of nursing homes and convalescent hospitals, loneliness, isolation, immobility, and fear of abandonment can become significant sources of anxiety and stress, as can the aging process itself. Long-term stress often leads to depression and to feelings of hopelessness and helplessness. Chronic stress can also engender exaggerated fears or explosive outbursts, for stress affects mental as well as physical states.

A person who becomes irritable and irrational from continued high level stress can pass this irritability on to others. This ripple effect is one of the many ways in which stress can affect a person's relationships as well as his or her physical body and mental well-being.

Receiving a diagnosis of a life-threatening illness, (or being closely related to someone who has received such a diagnosis) is listed close to the top of any list of stress-producing situations. The person who has been told that he or she has an incurable illness is faced not only with the immediate sense of loss of control, but with any number of concerns, decisions, anxieties, and fears. "How much time do I have left?" is often the first concern, followed by questions about what treatment course to follow, what the effects of the disease and/or treatment for the disease will be on mobility, life style, and quality of life. Anxiety over such issues as family finances, how to convey the news to family and friends, the ability of surviving family members to take care of themselves, how, where,and with whom to spend the rest of one's life can be highly stress-producing both for the person directly confronting the "terminal" illness and for family members and friends close to such a person.

Muscles contract under stress! When a muscle remains tense over a period of time, actual soreness in the muscle can result due to a build-up of lactic acid in the tissue. One does not have to be an athlete or a construction worker to develop sore muscles. Muscles can become tight and knotted from anxiety, fear, held-in sadness or anger, and even from thinking negative thoughts. A pattern emerges in which stress produces tension and discomfort, and that discomfort produces more stress.

Therapeutic massage can be a significant help in stress reduction and stress management for both the elderly and the ill. The massage therapy techniques employed in Compassionate Touch are effective in helping reduce muscular tension. As muscular tension disappears, anxiety is lessened, triggering a relaxation response, and overall stress is reduced. As tight muscles soften, tensions ease, and the mind and heart open, the person being touched may relax on deeper levels and begin to experience a sense of restful well-being.

It has been observed in intensive care units that even patients in a coma often appear to be more at peace after they are touched. Such patients register improved heart rate and brain waves when their hands are held. Individuals who are partially paralyzed and unable to speak, as the result of a stroke for instance, respond to touch in subtle but noticeable ways. Sometimes there is no visible movement or discernable recognition from such people, and yet often the jaw drops open, the eyes tear and/or the breathing pattern changes when Compassionate Touch is administered. I was once massaging the arms and hands of a woman who had been in a coma for several months when she suddenly took a deep breath followed by a long exhalation and sigh. It could have been coincidence, but I believe it was probably a response to the human contact and touch she was receiving.

Aid in Alleviating Depression

Anyone who works in long-term health care will tell you that depression is often a major problem among residents of nursing and convalescent homes. The malaise in some such facilities is almost palpable.

The less active elderly and/or the chronically ill are prone to periods of depression for a variety of reasons. As the aging process continues and/or an illness progresses, there may be ongoing or increasing physical limitations and discomfort. Change and loss are major components in frustration and stress, which can lead to depression. Consider the following list. Almost every resident of an extended care facility will be experiencing a good number of these changes and conditions:

- sensory impairment
- decreasing mobility
- functional limitations
- change in social status
- changes in relationships with children, friends, family members
- loss of home, familiar environment, community
- relocation
- reduction in personal space and belongings
- loss of meaningful work/activity
- loss of significant relationships, companionship
- loss of income
- loss of friends
- loss of spouse/sexual partner
- loss of personal identity/role
- loss of privacy
- loss of control over personal choices and life style habits

Some of these changes are inevitable in the aging process. Some may occur unexpectedly due to injury or illness. Regardless of the reasons, the changes in this list are significant ones and are likely to evoke feelings of vulnerability and powerlessness in the person who is experiencing them. The losses that occur as the aging process escalates often occur closer together, so that the person has less time to adjust to each event; and the changes tend to be more permanent than those that may occur in younger adulthood.

Those who are aging and/or ill—whether residing in a care facility, living with someone else, or still maintaining their own home—are likely to experience concern, anxiety or fear in regard to any number of the following issues:

- dependency on others
- financial security
- injury or illness
- cost of health care
- further physical and mental impairment
- physical discomfort, pain
- self-image
- victimization
- isolation, abandonment
- death and dying

Boredom, loneliness, isolation, feelings of becoming less and less "attractive" and more and more "useless" frequently lead to melancholia in the elderly and the ill. Unalleviated mental anxiety contributes to chronic depression.

Touch deprivation is a largely ignored yet major cause of depression among the elderly in our society. Attentive, nurturing touch can be a significant therapeutic factor in treating despondency in the aging and/or the ill because of its multiple psycho-social, mental, emotional, and physical benefits. Being stroked, held, gently massaged, and touched in a focused, unconditional way can draw a person out of isolation, help that person feel valued as a human being, and, quite literally, give him or her something to live for.

The continued need of the older person for loving touch is poignantly expressed in this portion of a poem by Donna Swanson found in *Images, Women in Transition* (St. Mary's College Press, 1977):

> *How long has it been since someone touched me*
> *Twenty years?*
> *Twenty years I've been a widow*
> *Respected,*
> *Smiled at,*
> *But never touched,*
> *Never held so close that loneliness*
> *was blotted out.*

The prescription for touch deprivation for the elderly, the ill, or for anyone, is really quite simple. The remedy is not time consuming, costly, or difficult. The results of treatment, which can be administered by almost any willing and caring person who is comfortable with hands-on caregiving, are easily identifiable, the effects sometimes immediately noticeable.

Increased Mobility

An increase in circulation and reduction in tension produced through the practice of various therapeutic massage techniques may well bring about an increase in mobility as well as a feeling of renewed strength or energy. A bedridden patient may be more inclined to feed himself or even to stand or walk with help after receiving massage therapy.

An increase in joint flexibility or range of motion may be noticed in smaller movements such as hand grasp strength or the ability of a person to reach out and pick up a cup of water or other object. One of my first Compassionate Touch clients was a nursing home resident in her late nineties who could no longer walk and spent most of her waking hours in a wheel-chair. Anna was a sweet, white-haired elderly lady with a beautiful smile, and she loved to have her hands massaged. One day, I noticed her watching me intently as I held one of her hands in both of mine and, using lotion and a gentle squeezing massage technique, worked slowly over her whole hand, stroking and manipulating each finger one by one. When I had completed the massage of each of her hands, she held her right hand up close to her face. She then began opening and closing her fingers in surprise and wonder, joyfully chuckling to herself and saying, "I didn't know I could do that!"

Experience of Being Nurtured and Cared For

Sensitive touch and gentle, caring, massage is one of the most relaxing and pleasant comfort measures we can provide for others, especially for those who may be experiencing touch deprivation as well as physical and emotional traumas. As a reassuring form of physical contact and communication, massage is a tangible act of caring. It not only feels good but it gives the receiver a sense of being nurtured, attended to, and cared for, which can affect the quality of that person's life considerably.

In the course of a long illness, which may include a variety of medical treatments and invasive procedures, people can begin to feel more like scrutinized objects than individuals. Those people experiencing temporary or permanent disfigurement or physical "abnormalities" may feel unattractive and sense that others are uncomfortable or embarrassed in their presence or are repelled by the sight of their bodies. The self-esteem of such people may begin to degenerate along with their bodies. Respectful, caring, attentive touch tells such people, in essence, that they are not ugly or untouchable, that they have value as human beings. If such touch is offered openly, lovingly, and non-intrusively, those people will be affected by another's willingness to touch them and by that person's desire to help ease their suffering. If the intention is pure and is directed toward the individual, the people will experience compassion and may begin to feel greater self-acceptance and self-worth. They may become more "at ease" or calm in regard to their physical problems and more accepting of their current situation. Compassionate Touch contributes not only to the receiver's physical comfort, but to an improved state of mind, emotional balance, and overall sense of well being.

Renewed Vitality

Many of the elderly people I see in retirement centers or convalescent facilities—especially those who receive few visitors—have fallen into a state of inertia due to extended inactivity and boredom. Hands-on care can help break this cycle. Therapeutic massage provides physical and mental stimulation by increasing the circulation of oxygen and the flow of blood throughout the body, including the brain. The one-on-one attention and human contact given in a Compassionate Touch session can boost self-esteem, and the verbal interaction may also stimulate brain activity. At the end of a session, recipients may feel more motivated to visit with roommates or, having received attention themselves, to give a bit of attention to someone else.

I have observed residents in nursing facilities suddenly "come alive"and begin moving, talking, and even singing after receiving the kind of caring support available to them through a Compassionate Touch session. I have also seen patients who were labeled as "troublemakers" or incessant "whiners" become sweet and docile when contacted through loving touch.

Recently I was moisturizing and massaging the hands of a long-time client of whom I am particularly fond. This gentle elderly woman was in a semi-comatose state the first time I met her, but, over the months, she has become more and more responsive to attention and touch. She occasionally ventures outside of her own private universe and speaks coherently in answer to a direct question, smiles sweetly, or makes some other kind of contact. On this particular day, she unexpectedly put one of her hands over mine and then began massaging my hands! This giving, interactive response on her part provided a wonderfully moving and memorable moment.

Therapeutic massage and touch administered over a period of time may accelerate the benefits to the receiver, yet even one short session can sometimes produce remarkable changes in a receptive patient. I once walked into a room in an extended-care facility and saw a pajama clad resident with no covers over him, curled up in a fetal position on his mattress. He had oxygen tubes in his nostrils, looked very uncomfortable, and seemed to be quite ill. I remember being somewhat reluctant to disturb this gentleman as he appeared to be sleeping, yet he had requested my services and his was the last name on my list of people to see that day. He was somewhat responsive to touch, though we never made eye contact, and he spoke very little during the twenty minutes or so I spent massaging his back and his extremities. Something about this man, whom I had never met before and whom I felt quite sure I would never see again, touched my heart. At the end of our session I told him quite honestly that I was very glad to have met him and to have spent a bit of time with him. I received a telephone call from the Activity Director of the facility the next day telling me that, much to her amazement, she had encountered the last gentleman I'd worked with out walking in the hallway asking when he could get another massage! He left to go home a few days later.

Emotional or Energy Release

Touch can act as a key to unlock "stuck energy" and emotions that have been denied or held in for months, even years, as most bodyworkers know. As a person experiences being accepted and cared for through loving touch, tense muscles begin to relax, and the heart begins to open, often allowing long repressed feelings to surface. Such emotional releases may be accompanied by trembling, shaking, laughter, or tears. There is almost always a deep sadness underlying an initial outburst of frustration or anger. The giver of Compassionate Touch can provide a significant service to another person in simply receiving such emotions as they come up, without evaluating or judging them. The person expressing long denied feelings or releasing withheld emotions may suddenly feel a lightening of the body, an increase in energy, and/or a renewed interest in actively relating to others.

One of my clients is a rather frail-looking woman in her eighties whom I see only once a month. She talks little but seems mentally aware and has a sweet and endearing smile. I usually moisturize and massage her hands and arms while she sits in her wheelchair in her room. Halfway through our first session, as I was stroking her upper arms with gentle pressure, she suddenly started shaking as a ripple of energy moved throughout her entire body and she exclaimed "Ooohhh, that feels sooooo good!" She continued to enjoy this energy release for several minutes, and the experience has been repeated almost every time I've seen her.

It is often easier for a person to communicate with someone with whom he or she has no particular role to fulfill in life, someone who does not have the expectations and attachments to that person that a family member has. Some people find it less difficult to share their deeper feelings with someone they have just met and may never see again than to talk about what they are experiencing with those who love them most.

I was once working with a middle-aged woman who I'd been told had suffered a stroke. As I began touching her feet, she stated that she'd had a bad fall. I did not comment except to say I was sorry. I continued massaging her foot and leg and then went on to the other foot. I felt her begin to relax a bit physically and, after a few more minutes, she made what was obviously to her a painful confession. "It wasn't a fall; I had a stroke." She then began to relax mentally as well as physically, and to trust me with the deeper truth of her experience and her fears about recovery.

The simplest acknowledgement of the reality of a situation can sometimes unleash a flood of emotion in a person who has few people to communicate with or who doesn't want to "burden" a family member. I remember well one not-so-elderly gentlemen in an extended care facility. On the list I was given of residents I would be seeing that day, his name had a notation beside it that he'd had both legs amputated in the past year. In the course of our conversation during his neck and shoulder massage, he mentioned that his wife had died less than a year ago. I observed that he had experienced a lot of loss in a short period of time, and he began to cry as he told me some of the details of those losses.

I was once asked to look in on a situation in which a widowed, wheelchair-bound mother in her seventies took a special van every afternoon from the assisted living center where she resided to an extended care facility in another town to sit with her son who lay, no longer able to speak, dying from AIDS. This woman had watched her other four children die from various unexpected accidents and diseases over the years. I could only begin to imagine what she must be experiencing and what a toll this situation was exacting on her body/mind. This woman had been told that therapeutic massage was available for residents of the facility but, according to the family services supervisor, she was highly resistant to the idea of anyone else touching her son.

I did not press this issue after introducing myself but instead began to gently massage her shoulders and upper back. She told me how wonderful it felt and how much she'd enjoyed the last massage she had received, seven years before during a hospital stay. She then rather abruptly wheeled her chair out into the hallway, indicating that she wanted me to follow her. She asked in somewhat urgent and hushed tones if I thought massage could actually help her son. I told her truthfully that it would not cure his disease or prolong his life but that it might help him to be more comfortable. She said rather dubiously, "let's try it once a month then, but I can't pay you today." I did not feel that her son would be alive in a month, or even in a week, and sensed that my only opportunity to work with him was probably the present moment, so I told her that immediate payment was not necessary and that I had some time available right then.

When I approached this once handsome and active man who I judged to be in his mid-thirties, he was clutching a large teddy bear, thrashing back and forth on the bed, twisting the sheets, and emitting a sound that could only be described as the kind of whimpering or whining cry a very frustrated and confused preschooler, grasping for control of his universe, would make. I placed one hand in the middle of his chest and touched his arm ever so gently and carefully, as I might a young child. He turned and looked directly at me for several moments, his body movement and whimpering stopped, and soon silent tears began to roll down his face. I said "It's all right," giving him the permission he perhaps could not give to himself with his mother watching, to release his tears. A few moments later, he suddenly turned over and, like an exhausted child, went right to sleep. To me, this incident was a clear example of the tremendous power of acceptance and acknowledgement.

Sense Memory

We all know what pleasure memories can bring. Receiving a massage can evoke pleasant memories of earlier times of being touched and the memory itself can trigger a relaxation response as well as bring pleasure to the person you are touching.

My services were once requested for a cancer patient who was experiencing a great deal of discomfort, particularly in her arms and shoulders. She was in the hospital the first time I visited her and was eager to be massaged. She was experiencing so much pain on that particular day, however, that even the softest touch on her upper arm or shoulder proved to be too much. (A large tumor growing in the upper node of one lung was pressing on a nerve and was apparently responsible for the shooting pains down her arm as well as the burning sensation she felt in her fingers.) This spirited 42-year old woman was very much awake and aware even though she was taking medication, including morphine, for her physical pain. Her condition reminded me of a woman's labor pains before birth, as the intense discomfort came upon her intermittently and demanded all her attention. She apparently noticed the similarity too, commenting wryly that dying of cancer was harder than giving birth.

I asked this patient if she would like a foot massage, to which she gave a resounding "Yes, I'd love that!" As I moved to the foot of the bed and began massaging her feet and legs, her husband, who was standing nearby, mentioned to me that his wife could no longer feel anything below the waist! I continued what I was doing, knowing that even though she couldn't feel my hands on her skin, the massage would help the circulation in her legs. What I didn't realize, until she told me, was that she enjoyed watching me massage her feet and legs because it helped her remember the pleasure which she and her husband had experienced in giving each other foot massages. She could also experience a slight sensation in her upper body when I held her feet and gently pulled. She even joked that I was "pulling her leg!"

Psycho-Social Benefits

For the institutionalized elderly, in particular, the psycho/social benefits of hands-on caregiving may be more significant and more immediately noticeable than the physical benefits. Such individuals may be given three "balanced" meals a day, yet they remain starved for companionship, for affection, and for meaningful social interaction.

A caring presence, reinforced by touch, offers relief from loneliness and isolation. It assuages feelings of abandonment and deprivation while offering reassurance, companionship, and support. It offers those who spend long hours deprived of meaningful human contact an opportunity to expand their focus by shifting their attention to something outside of their own minds. The physical interaction afforded by touch expands awareness; and the verbal interaction engages the mind in a different way, stimulating new mental activity and relieving boredom.

I remember reading of a nurse working with people suffering from dementia on a daily basis who said she considered touching to be a "first-class therapeutic tool." She greeted each person in her care with a handshake each morning, and she hugged each one in farewell before leaving the facility where she worked in the evening. This kind of conscious physical contact, no matter how brief, is a reminder and an affirmation to the one being touched that he or she is still alive, still part of the human race.

Touch is an excellent resource for caregivers and professionals alike in coping with challenging behaviors in those they care for. When persons suffering from dementia become disoriented and/or agitated, touch can be reassuring and calming, thus helping reduce apprehension and mental anxiety. Holding, gentle stroking, or even a firm hand grasp are kinds of touch that can be extremely useful in helping reorient or "ground" a person in present time and space. Touch is especially effective in helping someone to shift focus and/or regain equilibrium when it is combined with direct eye contact and with verbal information, such as telling a person his or her name, location, or what day it is.

As a form of direct, compassionate contact, touch can have an extremely powerful effect. The right kind of touch, given at just the right moment, can cut through the delusions of the mind like a sword through butter.

I feel sure that many of the people I see in extended care facilities and homes for the aged benefit as much from the conversations we have, and from being listened to, as they do from the touching they receive. I occasionally meet people who tell me initially that they do not like being touched, or that they don't "need" me, but who tolerate my presence, or a short back rub, because what they really want is human contact. They want someone to talk to. I never force hands-on work with such individuals, although in every case I can think of, the person's tolerance for touch has gradually increased to the point where he or she is able to derive pleasure from physical contact in some form. In the meantime, I might simply sit with the person and keep my attention on him or her. When someone understands that the contact I am offering is real and that it is unconditional, that person often begins talking and sharing all kinds of fascinating information about him or herself.

True listening is an active, learnable skill. It involves focusing one's attention, not just on what another person is saying, but on the individual who is talking. It involves putting aside one's own exterior and interior commentary in order to try to understand precisely what someone is communicating, listening not just to the words, but to the meaning behind the words and to the silences between words. Active listening means being open to another and focusing all one's available energy in the direction of that other person, doing one's best to understand and receive the real essence of what he or she is trying to communicate. It means patiently waiting and listening—with one's whole self. It is one of the greatest gifts we can give to another human being.

I have observed that the amount of attention many health care workers give to the individuals whom they serve is in direct proportion to the ability of the patient/resident to interact with them verbally and to comply with their instructions. Those who are less verbal or are combative in any way are avoided and sometimes even ignored. While this phenomenon is certainly understandable as a natural reaction, it serves to drive the less verbally responsive and less "cooperative" individuals further into isolation, depression, and, eventually, a "failure to thrive" syndrome.

It is my experience that most individuals who are labeled as "unresponsive" do respond to attentive touch, and to a caring human presence, in many subtle ways. It is important for those of us who relate to such individuals to continue developing in our ability to recognize these more subtle responses, and to develop the capacity to give the gift of our presence to another without expecting immediate compliance, feedback, or gratification.

I know of someone who, after completing a training course in working with the dying, went to her local convalescent hospital and volunteered to spend time with individuals in the facility who might be nearing death. After assuring my friend that there were no dying patients in her facility, the somewhat skeptical supervisor told my friend of a few people who weren't participating in any of the offered activities, or being visited by anyone else. My friend was drawn to one individual she found curled up in a fetal position on her bed in the last room at the end of a long hallway; so she simply sat beside this woman and consciously put her attention on her for 15-20 minutes each time she visited. Noticing that staff members who came into the room often talked about this resident as if she were not present, my friend always addressed the woman by her name. My friend knew intuitively that this woman was aware of her presence and of the attention she was giving her. Nothing dramatic, or measurable, happened, as it might in a movie, yet the woman eventually opened her eyes, there was real contact, and for those few moments at least, one "nonresponsive" resident of that facility knew that she was not alone.

Benefits for the Giver

I recently noticed a new title on the bookstore shelf, *The Healing Power of Doing Good*. Recent research is proving that helping others enhances one's own health, physically and psychologically. Dr. Herbert Benson, author of *The Relaxation Response*, has said that he might well prescribe volunteering as a way to reduce stress. The act of selfless giving can raise self-esteem, boost energy, help us lead more productive lives, and even add years to a lifetime.

Ancient wisdom also suggests that giving to others is a gift to the self. Jesus said that "It is more blessed to give than to receive." Eastern religion teaches that generosity and kindness to others brings the greatest happiness, purifying the heart and mind; and that inner tranquility and strength come from the development of love and compassion.

Hands-on nurturing care through massage heightens our sense of touch, makes us more sensitive to our own bodies, and helps us understand and acknowledge our own need for nurturing and love. It teaches us to treat ourselves, as well as others, with compassion.

Caring for others reminds us of how much we have to give, of what we can actually offer, to those with whom we share life's journey. Opening our hearts to others helps us identify ways in which we might ease the suffering of our fellow human beings, gives us the opportunity to experience our interdependence, and to experience the joy of service. Compassionate Touch provides us with a vehicle for service, an avenue for expressing our innate generosity, and a way of directly experiencing our kinship with others.

Choosing to be consciously *present with* and *attentive to* another creates a space for us to experience what is actually true in regard to that individual. When we follow our instinctive impulses to reach out in merciful kindness and care for another, we are acting from a level of beingness that is close to our own true nature. Any time we come out of our self-ness by deepening our contact with others, we have an opportunity to experience who we really are.

Being physically present with those who are in later life stages gives us a unique opportunity to confront our own mortality. It gives us a chance to look within and examine our resistances to life and our resistances to death. It gives us a chance to face our fears about living and about dying. Seeing someone ill and in pain reminds us that we could be that way too. It brings up thoughts of how it might be if and when we receive a "terminal" diagnosis. Will I be disfigured? Will I suffer horrible pain? Will I lose control of my bodily functions? Will I lose my hair or my eyesight or my ability to speak? Will I be a burden on my family? Will I become mentally incapacitated? Watching someone die makes us think of how we felt or how we may feel when someone we love dies. It makes us wonder what it will be like when we die. It helps us confront our attachments and our helplessness and it gives us the chance to greet our own pain and grief with mercy.

Administering Compassionate Touch teaches us how to be in the presence of suffering and to keep our hearts open instead of shutting down, turning away, or denying the pain we experience in ourselves and in others. In staying open we may experience the illusion of separateness dissolving.

The most significant benefit of practicing Compassionate Touch may be simply getting to know another human being. Any time we truly open our hearts to another individual, a part of who we are is reflected back to us and our vision is thus expanded. The personal bond that is created out of the intimate interaction in a Compassionate Touch session is of immeasurable benefit because it is always in the context of relationship that true healing and evolution occur.

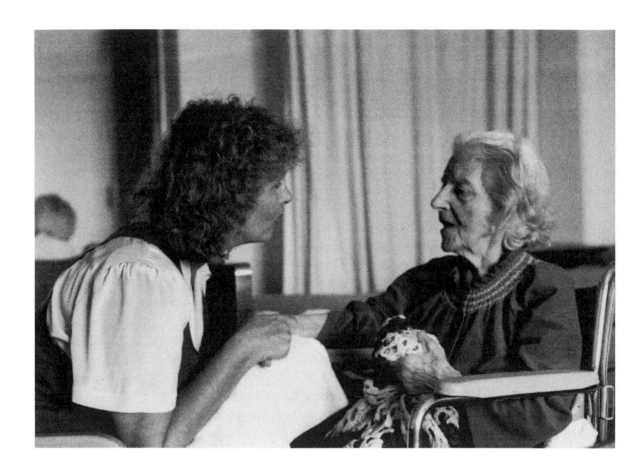

❧ 3 ❧

Characteristics and Abilities of the Compassionate Touch Practitioner

We cannot heal others, we can only heal ourselves so that our presence will be healing to others.

Irene Smith
Founder/Director of Service Through Touch

Those who spend a great deal of time caring for individuals who are elderly, ill, and/or dying, whether on a professional or volunteer basis, are probably caring and sensitive people. Caregivers are usually motivated, for a variety of reasons, to be of service to their fellow human beings. They most likely possess some or all of the characteristics and abilities discussed in this chapter.

One should at least have an interest in and a potential for developing these abilities in order to become a successful practitioner of Compassionate Touch. It is not necessary to be a professionally trained and/or licensed massage therapist in order to practice hands-on caregiving, though such knowledge and experience would certainly be useful. Since whatever natural or learned abilities we possess will continue to develop with practice, mastery of any skill should be seen as a long-term project.

Touch Oriented

Though it may seem too obvious to mention, an interest in communicating through physical contact is the first characteristic that a practitioner of Compassionate Touch needs to have. Not everyone is interested in or good at connecting with others in a "hands-on" physical way. Some people are especially skilled at "reaching out and touching" another person through words. They are particularly good at eliciting an emotional or mental response through what they say and how they say it. Those same people may have no particular desire or interest in communicating through physical contact. To practice Compassionate Touch, it is important to have some facility for tactile contact. You need to have a desire to make contact with another in a physical way and be willing to develop your skills in this type of relating.

Intuitive

To be intuitive means to be able to perceive or become aware of something through a source other than the thinking mind or the senses. When you simply understand or know a thing without going through any intellectual or logical process to come to that understanding, you are using an internal system of perception known as your intuition.

The ability to access your own inner wisdom will be of great value in practicing Compassionate Touch. Using your intuition becomes particularly important when a person can no longer communicate verbally or reasonably with you or when you are working with someone who speaks a different language than the one you speak. Working intuitively and in contact with each individual, you will eventually know what part of the body to touch as well as when and how to touch it. You will know when to listen and when to speak. You will automatically act appropriately and accurately in most situations. This intuitive ability might be referred to as following your feelings, listening to your inner voice, listening with your heart, or sensing what is best, as opposed to thinking too much about what to do or coming to a logical decision. Cultivating a connection with "the teacher within," and learning to follow this inner guidance gives you access to a valuable reservoir of information that can be of great help to you in working with others.

An intuitive leap can occur when the mind is confronted with something that it cannot easily grasp or assimilate. In this sense, working with those who are critically, or chronically ill, disabled and/or near death gives you the opportunity to become more familiar with your intuitive nature. It is your intuition, as well as your compassion, that will allow you to sense the innermost fears and thoughts of another. As your heart opens to what your mind may not easily absorb, you will rely more on your intuitive wisdom to reveal to you what to say or not to say, how to touch or not to touch in any given moment.

Able to Adapt

Compassionate Touch sessions are given to people in a wide variety of situations and under constantly changing conditions. It is essential for the practitioner to be comfortable working in different ways with different people, as well as in different ways with the same person. As a Compassionate Touch caregiver, you must be able to adjust quickly and easily to the environment as well as to the changing physical, psychological, and mental states of the people you work with. You will encounter people who are physically connected to all kinds of medical equipment and apparatus. You will be working with people exhibiting varying degrees of alertness and coherence of thought as well as varying degrees of physical and psychological pain. You will be seeing people whose condition can change drastically from day to day, even hour to hour. You may be touching a person in her or his last hour or minute of life. You need to develop the ability to stay consciously present from moment to moment, whatever occurs. You must be able to drop your preconceived ideas and thoughts about making things be different than they actually are, so that your actions are appropriate to each individual and to each situation as it unfolds.

There is an element of unpredictability any time you are interacting with human beings in crisis. Offering support and relief to those who are seriously ill and/or in later life stages challenges you to remain flexible and adaptable. Such a practice offers you many opportunities to be spontaneous and creative.

Open-Hearted

It is essential for the Compassionate Touch practitioner to be open and receptive. The heart must expand to include that which is not only new and different, but also frightening, possibly even terrifying, to the mind. It is useful to have the quality of "seeing" with your heart, and with all of your senses, when working with the aged, the seriously ill, and with those who are nearing death.

Opening your heart to another leaves you vulnerable and unprotected in a certain sense. You cannot really open to another without also being open to your own feelings of sadness, fear, loneliness, and anger. Choosing to be open brings you closer to those whom you want to serve and, at the same time, opens the door into your own subconscious. Your openness will bring your own fears into the light of consciousness and perhaps into expression, so that they can no longer be denied.

Your openheartedness will bring reality into your hands-on caregiving sessions and into your relationships with the people you touch. Opening your mind and heart to the individual whom you are touching, being with that person just as he or she actually is, and surrendering your ego in service to that individual can significantly affect your life.

Sense of Self

Being well grounded in the reality of your own being is an important quality for a practitioner of hands-on caregiving to possess. In other words, you need to have a conscious awareness of your own physical presence, a clear sense of your physical and psychological boundaries.

One reason this sense of self is important is that without it you may find that you begin identifying with the people with whom you are working to the point of "merging" with them emotionally, mentally, or energetically. While this is an interesting metaphysical exercise, it is not, ultimately, the best way to serve others in the context of administering Compassionate Touch.

If you are not a person who always feels naturally "grounded," or physically connected to the earth, it may be useful for you to practice bringing your attention and awareness to your physical being. I use the following exercise to remind myself of the simple fact that I am in a physical body walking on the earth and supported by it. (It is also a good technique to use when you "fly off the handle" and want to "come back to earth.")

> *Close your eyes and bring your attention inside your body. Inhale deeply through both of your nostrils and then exhale through your mouth. As you exhale, feel the density of your physical body as you sit or stand on solid ground. Become conscious of the reality of your body in contact with the solid matter of the earth. Feel the earth supporting your physical presence on it. To carry this grounding exercise further, imagine an invisible but impermeable pole extending from deep within the center of the earth, coming up through the surface of the ground and into your body. Visualize this pole coming up through the center of your body and out through the top of your head, extending up into infinity. Continue breathing and being consciously aware of your body in contact with the earth itself.*

Another aid in experiencing a sense of self is the ability to remain centered or in touch with your own inner energy source. Here is one simple centering exercise:

> *Close your eyes and breathe deeply into your belly. Find the place inside that feels like the center of your physical being. It may be near your navel or lower in your body or it may even be around the area of your heart. Continue your abdominal breathing and keep your awareness inside your own body until you feel calm and centered within. Keep your attention on your breathing as you inhale and exhale. You may want to imagine a bright light or an energy source originating in the center of your physical being and radiating outward through all parts of your body, including your hands and fingertips.*

Try to take a few moments, before entering the home or the room of a person with whom you are about to work, to let go of the outside world and to get in touch with yourself so that you can be fully present during each Compassionate Touch session.

Able to Focus Energy

The ability to keep your attention and your energies directed toward one person or one thing at one time is a useful skill to possess in any endeavor. In fact, it is difficult to accomplish anything without focus!

In the area of bodywork and massage, it is necessary to maintain focus in two ways. Keeping your attention or focus on the person with whom you are working is one way. In other words, you need to develop the ability to put aside any distractions that might take your attention away from the person you are touching. Distractions could be anything from your own mental thoughts about the person's physical condition, to an aide using a vacuum cleaner in the hallway of a nursing home. One distraction comes from within and the other from the environment.

Your own thoughts and feelings can splinter your attention in subtle and almost imperceptible ways. You may be the kind of person who can think about or do several things at the same time and so you find you are planning what to prepare for a family dinner while you are giving a foot massage to an elderly woman in her hospital bed. Although it looks the same to an observer, this experience is not the same, for the elderly woman or for you, as the experience of keeping your attention focused completely and only on the individual whom you are touching. You can experience the difference for yourself by doing the following exercise with a friend or loved one:

> *Put your attention on your friend and take one of his or her hands between your own two hands. As you hold your friend's hand begin to consciously apply a gentle, squeezing pressure. You do not have to look into the eyes of your friend while doing this, but do keep your attention solely on her or him. Continue to massage, sensitively and gently, the hand which you are holding, and then move on to the fingers, carefully going over each one and keeping your attention focused on your friend. When you have attentively touched and massaged the whole hand, place it carefully on your friend's lap. Now begin thinking about something else or looking around the room to see what you can see. Without putting your attention on your friend or what you are doing, just reach over and casually pick up your friend's other hand. Touch and stroke it while you continue thinking about something else unconnected in any way with what you are doing. Now, ask your friend to tell you what*

he or she experienced and how each hand feels at this point. Switch roles so
that you can experience being the recipient of touch which is, at first, focused
in a conscious, attentive way and then given in an off-hand and random way.

You may experience a dramatic change when the attention of the person massaging you shifts away from being totally focused on you, or you may only notice a subtle difference the first time you try this exercise. Notice what it is like for you to touch someone else with focused attention and then to touch that person with your attention wandering or on something else entirely.

The second kind of focus that is useful in the practice of therapeutic massage is the ability to direct your energy in a physical way. In other words, you want to be able to willfully channel your energy in a specific direction, or at least be able to allow the life-force to flow out of your body and through your hands to another. Practice the following exercise when you want to remind yourself of the reality of this energy or refocus your attention on experiencing the energy that emanates out from your physical body:

While sitting or standing, make sure that you feel both grounded and
centered within yourself. Then bring your open hands together in front of
your body and rub the palms together quickly until you feel heat. Now,
focus your attention on the palms of your hands and very slowly move
your hands a little apart from each other, then slowly bring the palms
closer together again. Notice what occurs or what feelings you experience
as you do this. Practice moving your hands even further apart and notice
at what point you feel a change in the sensation or connection between
your two hands. You can do a similar exercise with a friend, putting your
two open hands in front of you with the palms facing the palms of the
other person. Experiment with focusing your attention on experiencing
the energy field that builds up between your sets of hands as you move
them closer together and then further apart.

When you put your attention on your own life-force or energy, you may experience it as a tingling sensation or perhaps as something like an electrical current moving through your body, or as heat or light or pulsation. You may experience the energy flowing inside and/or just outside your body. Once you have focused your attention on this energy and experienced it, you can experiment with consciously directing it. As you breathe from your center, you can practice letting the energy move and into your arms, down into your hands, and out through your fingers.

As you concentrate on focusing and directing your energy, you will notice that this skill eventually becomes automatic. You may feel it more intensely at times or moving through you in different ways, but you will no longer have to think about it each time you begin to touch someone.

Willing to Face Death

Gay Luce, a prominent teacher in the field of death and dying, says that we put much more time and energy into getting ready for a trip to Hawaii than we do in preparing for our own death. This is particularly true in our Western culture where the fact of death is often hidden and denied as long as possible.

An important characteristic for the Compassionate Touch practitioner to possess is something I would call Death Awareness or Death Preparation. You need to have confronted, to some degree, your own fears about death and dying. You need to have accepted the fact of your own mortality and to have the conscious awareness that death is a natural part of the life-cycle and that you and everyone you love will one day die.

It will be helpful for you, as a Compassionate Touch practitioner, to have identified what your areas of concern are in relation to death and dying, to have some awareness of, and some experience in, processing your own fears about death. By processing I mean opening your mind and heart to let your thoughts, concerns, and fears about death and dying surface. I mean examining those fears until you have at least some understanding of where they come from or what they are based on. I mean communicating those fears to others verbally and possibly in other ways, such as through writing or art. Part of your process may be, or may become, consciously confronting your own fears by being around or working with those who are manifesting what you fear most.

One technique I use for accessing thoughts and feelings that I have not yet brought to conscious awareness is to do a dyad exercise. I ask a trusted friend or colleague to do the exercise with me. We decide on a topic and on a specific instruction to be given such as "Tell me a concern you have about aging," or "Tell me a fear you have about dying." We decide on the amount of time we will spend doing the exercise (thirty to forty minutes is a good time frame) and make a commitment to stick with the exercise for that length of time. A watch or timer can be set to signal the end of the period.

Here are the steps for doing such an exercise if you want to try it:

1. Sit down opposite another person in chairs, or on pillows on the floor facing each other, a comfortable distance apart but not touching.
2. Decide on a specific instruction and stick with that wording throughout the exercise.
3. Decide which person will talk first and which person will listen first.
4. The person designated as the first listener then gives the instruction to his or her partner. For example: "Tell me a concern you have about aging."
5. The other person receives the instruction, puts his or her full attention on that instruction, and then notices what occurs. That person then

communicates verbally to his or her partner whatever came up as a result of that focus. The person is to include thoughts, feelings, emotional reactions—whatever occurred in the body/mind.

6. The listening partner remains open to the other person and to receiving what that person is communicating, without interacting verbally or physically, and without evaluating or judging anything that is said.

7. When the communicating partner has gotten across what actually occurred in his or her consciousness as a result of receiving and contemplating that particular instruction—no more and no less—the listening partner says: "Thank You," or something similar, to acknowledge the communicating partner for responding to the instruction, and to indicate that the communication has been received.

8. The roles then reverse and the person who has been communicating gives the same instruction to his or her partner.

9. The exercise continues in this way until the end of the agreed upon time period.

This kind of exercise can be a powerful and effective tool in accessing and processing thoughts and feelings. The exercise also serves to improve your communication skills and to deepen your contact with others. You can use this type of dyad exercise to work on almost any issue or area of life in which you feel "stuck," to help you move forward.

Once you have begun this self-examination process in regard to illness, aging, death, and dying, it will simply continue and deepen through your service to others. You may well encounter new fears as you continue to work with people (when you see someone your own age unable to speak or move, or a child suffering intense physical pain, for example). If you have developed some facility for facing and accepting your fears as they arise, then you will be able to keep your attention on the individual you are working with when your own anxiety and fears are awakened during a session. You can notice and acknowledge, rather than repress or ignore, your reaction and go on with your session anyway. After the session you can look more closely at your responses and examine them. This process will begin to unfold more easily and more quickly until you hit a barrier, some new and previously denied personal experience with death (your own parent dying suddenly or a friend's child drowning, for example). Once you have confronted that particular barrier and moved through it, then you will simply continue your personal growth on a deeper level.

If you are working with the frail elderly or with other individuals who are nearing the end of their lives, it may be helpful for you to have some knowledge of the signs and symptoms of approaching death (see Appendix I). You may be working with an individual as that person approaches this transition. You may actually be the only one present as that person breathes his or her last breath. The more acceptance and understanding you have of the death experience, the more support you can offer. You will be able to remain calm and alert, and keep your attention on the individual as you witness such a moment.

Stephen Levine said, in a workshop I once attended, that being with another human being at the moment of his or her death is a rare and wonderful opportunity, an experience to be welcomed, because there is much to learn from sharing in and witnessing such a significant event. I have found his statement to be profoundly true. I heard another teacher speak recently about feeling excited, even elated, each time he is called upon to be with someone who is dying, because he knows he is going to be in the presence of Truth.

Able to Focus on the Individual

The ability to put your attention on another person as an individual is one of the most useful skills you can have in relating to those in later life stages. It will, in fact, help you greatly in all relationships.

With practice you can develop your capacity to see beyond a disabled, disfigured, or decaying body, to see beyond a cranky or argumentative personality. You can develop the ability to keep your attention on the individual rather than on an agitated mind or a painful physical condition. With practice, you can begin to de-identify the individual, not only from his or her body but from states of being or from particular points of view that are being expressed. It is useful to notice that points of view, mental states, emotional states, and physical conditions all change. Yet the individual exists and is there throughout the changes that the body or the mind goes through.

Noticing a person's state of mind and the physical condition of the body that person inhabits, especially when you are about to touch the body, is important. If, however, your attention stays focused only on a person's suffering, physical condition, or anxieties, you will be less able to serve that individual. You will be trying to contact that person through your reactive mind rather than from a centered, focused, and balanced state of consciousness.

I am not suggesting that you should be blind to, or unaffected by, the pain or suffering of those you care for. I am saying that the most compassionate thing and the most conscious thing that you can do is to notice your reaction to the person's condition and then put your thoughts aside in order to be present with the individual who is in that condition or state.

I once volunteered to massage a man who had been suffering for nearly fifteen years from a rare neuromuscular disorder. This particular disease causes severe, involuntary muscular contractions in the body, usually in the shoulders, the neck, and the face. In this person's case, the right shoulder was in continuous spasm and the head was being pulled to one side by constant and irregular jerking movements in the neck. As a result of this constant movement, the man's jaw had been pulled out of alignment, which affected his speech and made it difficult to decipher what he was saying. The progression of the disease had eventually made swallowing so difficult that his entire diet was in liquid form and was given to him through a gastrotomy tube, as were all his medications. He used a machine, much like those that dentists use, to aspirate saliva when it collected in his mouth. He had developed the habit of holding a small handkerchief over his face and mouth or between his lips. This was partially to hide his face from visitors, perhaps to alleviate their discomfort and embarrassment, as well as his own, and also to keep his teeth from biting into his lips. This person's muscle spasms were more or less violent from day to day, and he sometimes had a continuous tick near one eye, which gave him the feeling that there was some small object in the eye causing incessant irritation. His urine was passed through a catheter and collected in a bag hooked to the side of his bed. An oxygen tank and mask, as well as an IV stand, stood ready beside his bed.

I had never met anyone with this particular disease or in this type of ongoing predicament. I felt somewhat overwhelmed with the sight that greeted me as I walked to this gentleman's bedside. A number of thoughts and feelings arose in me as I began touching him. I felt great sadness for him and for his wife. I felt fear that I or somebody I loved could suddenly be afflicted with a disease such as this person suffered from. I wondered how I would cope with such a tragedy. I felt a bit guilty that this person had been in such a helpless physical state for so many years while I was healthy and actively walking around. I was filled with a desire to "help" this person, to "do" something to alleviate his pain and suffering.

Instead of taking a moment to notice and acknowledge my reactions to the situation and then give my attention to the person who was bedridden and disabled by this unusual disease, I tried to ignore my emotions, override everything I was thinking, and administer massage therapy. I wasn't centered and I wasn't really relating to this man as an individual; I was in a mental daze and simply "going through the motions." Consequently, I came away from my first visit with this gentleman somewhat numb and, eventually, in physical and emotional discomfort myself. If that person had died before our next session I would never have known him. I would have remembered only a body in pain, rather than the miraculously pleasant, loving, and gracious man who inhabited that body. It was a dramatic lesson for me and one that I have never forgotten.

The following lines were taken from a publication by Laguna Honda Hospital. They were written by a woman in the geriatric ward of the Hospital and discovered in her locker, after she died, by staff members who thought she was incapable of writing . . .

What do you see, what do you see?
What are you thinking when you are looking at me?
A crabbed old woman, not very wise
Uncertain of habit, with faraway eyes
Who dribbles her food and makes no reply.
When you say in a loud voice, "I do wish you'd try."
I'll tell you who I am as I sit here so still,
I'm a small child of ten with a father and mother
Brothers and sisters who love one another;
A bride soon at twenty, my heart gives a leap
Remembering the vows that I promised to keep
At twenty-five now I have young of my own
Who need me to build a secure happy home.
At fifty once more babies play round my knee
Again we know children, my loved ones and me.
Dark days are upon me, my husband is dead
I look to the future and I shudder with dread
My young are all busy rearing young of their own
And I think of the years and the love I have known.
I'm an old woman now and Nature is cruel
Tis her jest to make old age look like a fool.
The body crumbles, grace and vigour depart
There is now a stone where I once had a heart.
But inside this old carcass a young girl still dwells
And now and again my battered heart swells
I remember the joys; I remember the pain
And I'm loving and living all over again.
And I think of the years all too few . . . gone too fast
And accept the stark fact that nothing will last
So open your eyes, open and see,
Not a crabbed old woman; look closer . . . see me

If you focus your attention on someone's physical condition, illness, or state of being, you will miss a unique opportunity to meet and relate to that individual. Compassionate Touch is not hands touching or massaging a body, but a relationship between one individual and another!

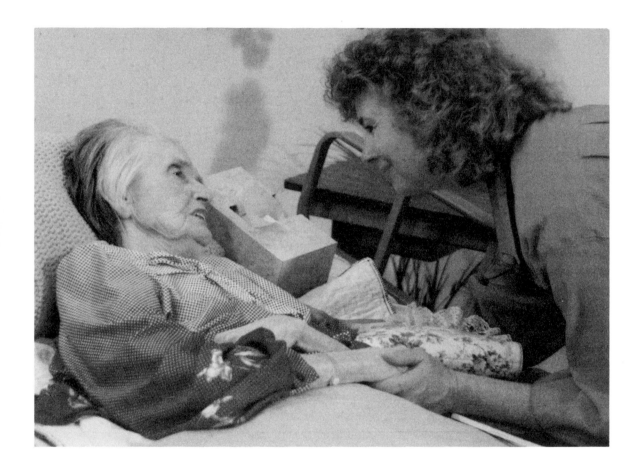

❦ 4 ❦

Useful Tools

A seeker of Truth: "How do I find God?"
The teacher: "Feed people."
Seeker: "How do I get enlightened?"
Teacher: "Serve people."

Ram Dass

The qualities of character and the abilities discussed in Chapter Three are the most important tools for the practitioner of Compassionate Touch. Those innate qualities and the willingness to develop your skills are essentially all that you need to begin. There are, however, a few practical items that can be helpful when used as aids in conjunction with your inner resources and abilities. If you are a home caregiver you might want to gather some of these items together and keep them in one place so that they are handy when you need them. If you are giving Compassionate Touch sessions as an outreach service, you can use a special tote bag to hold the items you may need, and take the bag with you when you go out to give sessions.

Oils and Lotions

Many Compassionate Touch techniques can be done without the use of oil, which is often unnecessary or inappropriate. In some situations and for certain techniques, however, some kind of lubricant is needed. (The specific uses of oils and lotion in administering Compassionate Touch will be addressed in Chapter Five.)

The best thing to do is to carry some massage oil and some lotion with you to each Compassionate Touch session so that you will have them if needed. There are many kinds of oils and lotions on the market touted as the perfect massage product. Some are quite expensive, difficult to find and, contain various additives. Some can be purchased in any grocery store.

Professional bodyworkers and their clients often develop a preference for one kind of lubricant or another. I have had regular massage therapy clients bring their own oil because it contained a scent they particularly liked or because it had been advertised to have special healing qualities or effects. I personally prefer vegetable oils to mineral oils (including baby oil) for the simple reason that repeated use of mineral oil clogs the pores. I feel that vegetable oils are healthier for the skin. Almond oil and apricot kernel oil are good. You can also use the less expensive safflower oil. I like to use coconut oil, which is light and natural with only a hint of scent. Coconut oil absorbs easily into the skin and does not turn rancid on sheets or clothing. It can be purchased in health food stores. At first glance, this product looks very much like mayonnaise since it comes in a wide mouth glass jar and is white when solidified. You need to heat the jar and then funnel the liquefied oil into a plastic squeeze-top bottle. (You can purchase these types of containers in health and beauty sections of drug or variety stores.) Unless the weather is exceptionally warm, you will need to liquefy the oil again before each use. You can do this by placing the plastic bottle in a microwave for about one minute, or by letting the bottle sit in very hot water in a small bowl or pan for a few minutes. Heating coconut oil converts it into a usable liquid form and gives the added comfort of warmth when applied to the skin. If you do not have use of a microwave oven (nursing homes and hospitals may or may not allow you access to their microwave) and if hot water is not readily available, you can quickly convert a small amount of the oil by simply rubbing it between the palms of your hands.

Lotion may be used to reduce friction during massage in the same way you would use oil. Which lubricant you choose to use is simply a matter of preference for you and for the person you are massaging. If your goal is primarily to moisturize dry skin, then lotion is a better choice than oil. Hospitals sometimes supply lotions to patients, but I have found that those lotions tend to be "sticky" and not the best for use in massage, so I always take my own lotion when visiting someone in a medical or extended care facility.

It is best to use oils and lotions without added fragrance whenever possible, unless the person you are working with makes a specific request. Some older people have a heightened sense of smell and find strong scents overpowering or unpleasant. Those who are ill are often particularly sensitive to odors and may feel temporary aversions to certain fragrances that did not bother them in the past. This may be especially true of people who are undergoing radiation or chemotherapy treatments.

If you discover particularly dry skin on the hands or feet, you may want to use a heavier body lotion in that area, or perhaps a cream such as Eucerine, which can be purchased in drug or grocery stores. Be on the lookout for unusually dry or cracked skin, especially around elbows or knees and on the feet and legs.

Try out a few oils and lotions to discover which you feel most comfortable using. In general, look for oils that are not heavily scented and contain more natural than artificial ingredients. I have found that mixing lotion with a small amount of oil works well and I usually use the combination in massaging the elderly. Lotion is more familiar to people and is easier to extract and apply. If someone you are working with has his or her own lubricant, or makes a special request that you are able to comply with, then by all means use what that person chooses.

Other Aids

Powder applied to the skin can feel soothing and comforting. Some people may prefer it to the feel of lotion or oil on their skin. Dry powder is easily applied and, perhaps because of its association with babies and mothering, can contribute to a feeling of being nurtured and taken care of. It is a good idea to apply powder to areas of the body that tend to collect moisture or do not get exposure to air, such as underneath large breasts, between the buttocks, or between the toes. There may be times when you will want to use powder for specific problems, as an alternative to a moisturizer, or just for a change. Cornstarch base powders are preferable to talc if there is any chance of a patient breathing talc into the lungs. A sample or travel size container of powder will last for some time.

A few small hand towels can prove quite useful during a Compassionate Touch session. You can roll up a towel (or towels) and put it under an ankle to elevate a foot or arm for easier access, or to allow for better circulation. You can spread the towel across your lap before resting an arm or leg on top of it. The towel can also be helpful in keeping the lubricant you are using off your clothing. You might use the towel for wrapping around a foot to warm it or for removing any excess oil that has not been absorbed into the skin. I have used a towel over the bedside rail or a wheelchair arm for help in gripping as well as for comfort. A towel can also come in handy if someone happens to begin vomiting while you are massaging him or her and a suitable container is not easily accessible nearby.

A small tubular-shaped neck pillow can also be a helpful accessory. Some patients like it as a change from the larger bed pillow or you can use it to give added support to a person's neck by putting it on top of the bed pillow. If you are standing behind a desk chair or wheel chair, you can put the pillow between the patient's neck and your body and let the person relax against it. If someone's head falls to one side or the other, the pillow can be used for support between the head and the shoulder. The neck pillow can also provide support under an ankle or knee while you are working. It is more easily negotiated than a large bed pillow, which may or may not be available.

Another item I usually carry with me is a small jar of Tiger or Dragon Balm. I would not use such a product routinely or even very often, but it can be quite effective in soothing accumulated muscular tension in the shoulder and back area, or muscles in a state of spasm or contraction. Tiger Balm is an analgesic salve, manufactured in Singapore and easily obtainable in health food stores or herbal pharmacies. It contains camphor and menthol as well as peppermint, cassia and clove oils. The milder version is white in color while the extra strong salve is a reddish orange. Both strengths do have a strong scent and I would never use this kind of product without asking a patient if it was acceptable or without explaining its use and effect. It feels much the same on the skin as "Deep Heat" or other old fashioned type liniments. A person's skin will feel noticeably tingly and warm soon after Tiger Balm is applied. Never use Tiger Balm near open sores, on damaged skin, or near any body orifice. Clean the Balm off your hands after using it and before going on to massage other parts of the body!

You might want to keep with you a small container (not a roll up tube) of salve or balm for applying to parched and chapped lips. Eucerine can also be applied for this purpose. One caregiver I know, whose husband was unable to take even liquids by mouth for several years, said Eucerine was the best thing she ever found for preventing chapped lips. If the patient needs assistance, use your fingertip to apply the salve and remember to wash your hands before and after such applications if you will be using the same container with another patient.

You may want to carry a small container of microbial soap such as Betadine (purchased in a drug store) with you. A few moist towelettes, such as you might use in the car and on camping trips, can also come in handy in case soap and water are not readily available.

 I have found it useful to wear an apron with pockets (such as those worn by waiters or beauticians) when working on a number of individuals consecutively. The apron protects clothing and provides a place to keep containers of lotion and other small items so that they are easily accessed as needed. Such aprons can be made or bought in a variety of colors and materials. There is also a product on the market called a massage holster—something similar to a carpenter's belt except that it has only one or two loops for carrying bottles of lotion or oil. If you are standing up, a pump-type bottle of lotion fitted into such a belt frees the hands and allows easy and quick access to the lubricant as you work.

It is good to keep some latex or vinyl gloves handy (in a pocket or bag) just in case they are needed (see Chapter Six for a discussion of when to wear gloves). Oil can break down the surface of gloves, so it would be best to use a water-based lotion if you need a lubricant while working with gloves on. In any case, once they have been worn, the gloves should be discarded.

Whether you are seeing people as a professional massage therapist or a volunteer caregiver, it is good to wear a name badge, or at least an identification sticker, so that people will know who you are and what you do. Seeing your name in writing as well as hearing it will help people to remember it. An identification badge may be especially appreciated by individuals who are hard of hearing and/or nonverbal.

None of these items is absolutely essential for administering massage or attentive touch. I have found frequent uses for most of them during Compassionate Touch sessions, however, and I like to have them with me to expand my options. They all fit easily into a medium size canvas tote bag, which you can keep in your car or near your front door so that it is easily accessible whenever you need it.

Music

Music seems to have a special power to affect consciousness, and sound can have a profound effect on the nervous system. The ancient Greeks believed that music could be used to heal. They played zithers as an aid to digestion and played other instruments to induce sleep and to treat mental disturbances. Many contemporary practitioners of holistic health care use music in working with clients as part of the therapeutic process. There are several books on the market today that address this experience in detail.

It is clear that certain kinds of music can enhance the relaxation experience, though the same music does not work with every person. If you sense that listening to some soft or calming music might be helpful to someone you are massaging, do not hesitate to suggest playing it, either during or after your session with that person. Although music is not an integral part of a Compassionate Touch session, it can contribute to and enhance the relaxation process, and it is not likely to be detrimental in any way.

I have, on occasion, brought a cassette tape recorder and tape with me to a session and played some music in working with a particular person. One gentleman I work with who is blind likes to listen to tape recordings of certain kinds of music. I have found that he becomes more relaxed, less distracted, and more open to touch when I put on a Benny Goodman or a Jimmy Dorsey tape during our sessions.

I once visited a patient I'd been working with for some weeks; he was growing increasingly weak and was preparing to die. This man was an accomplished musician. On this particular day, his caregiver had put on a tape recording of a pianist playing as beautifully as anyone I've ever heard. As I sat with this individual, touching him softly, and breathing with him in those precious moments, the sweetness of the music seemed to fill the room and enfold us until it felt as if we both disappeared inside of the sound. It was an experience I will never forget. While listening to his favorite opera a few days later, this gifted, gentle man slipped quietly out of his body as the recording he was listening to reached its last act climax.

Occasionally, people may find music, even recordings that they previously requested or enjoyed, to be unpleasant or irritating. In later life stages, some people's hearing becomes acutely sensitive and they may find almost any sound, including those that may once have been soothing and enjoyable, an annoyance. Even talking, at some stage, can become jarring to the psyche. It is best just to sit quietly with people who are in this state, maintaining contact and touching them in whatever way seems most appropriate.

Other people nearing death may become oblivious to sound, simply "tuning out" everything except what they want or need to hear. Some elderly or quite ill people begin making their own special sounds. This may be a plea for more attention, or it may be a means of self-expression or self-comfort. For some weeks before my grandmother died, she frequently made a continuous humming sound, almost like a chant. Before this time she had often enjoyed hearing me sing to her or listening to a tape of me singing or reading. At this point, however, it seemed to me that she was making her own music, so to speak, and that to impose other sounds on her would be intrusive and disruptive. It was obvious that the sound she was making was comforting to her, and it seemed to be happening spontaneously. I have occasionally walked into convalescent hospitals and heard a virtual chorus of singing, chanting, and "sounding" from residents.

Respect the individual at all times, give the person you are working with as much control as possible, and do what you can to honor him or her during the time you are together. You cannot change the script of a person's life nor can you prevent death, but you may be able to contribute to an improved quality of life or to help someone die with a measure of dignity, supported by human contact.

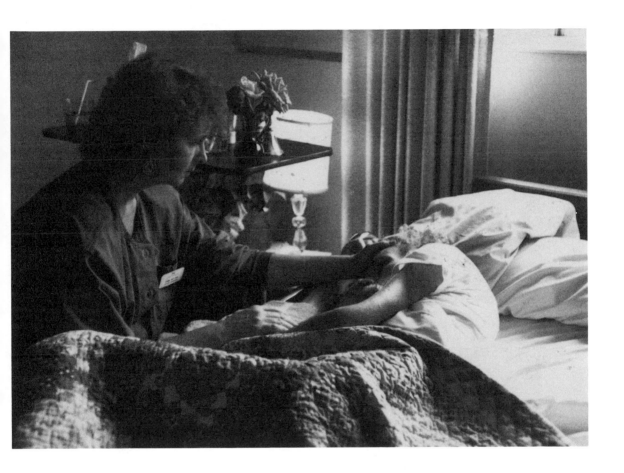

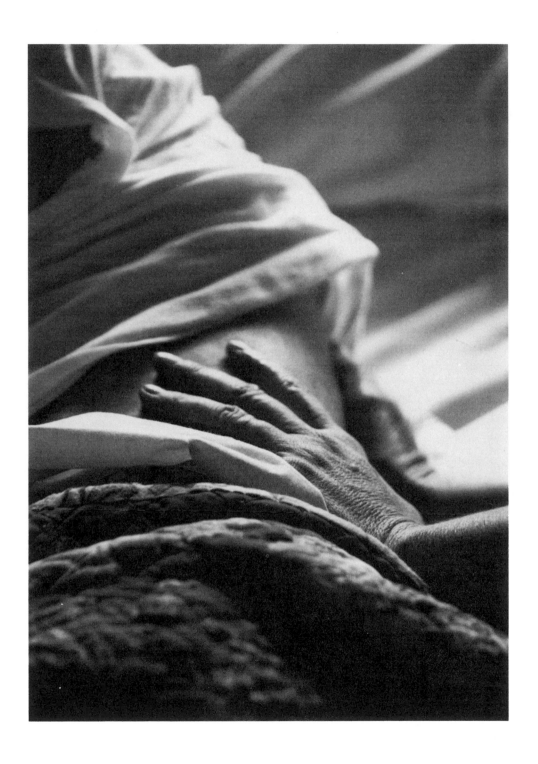

❧ 5 ❧

Compassionate Touch
Techniques

Do unto others as you would have them do unto you.

Jesus of Nazareth

The ability to truly put your attention on the individual whose body you are touching is more important than any specifically learned techniques. If you develop the ability to "see" an individual rather than just looking at a body, and if you reach out to that individual with a caring and open heart, your touch is likely to be far more effective than that of a highly trained professional who may be simply going through the mechanics of manipulating a physical body. Out of your real and pure contact with the individual, you will intuitively know what to do and how to proceed.

Knowledge of particular ways of touching and of administering massage is useful, however, in building confidence and in expanding options. Learning a few simple techniques will give you a base from which to build as well as some practical skills for use in combination with your natural "knowing" and your intuitive sense.

If you have already studied a particular form of massage therapy or bodywork or are a professional practitioner, then working with the aging and the ill will simply require adapting whatever method or systems you already know and use to a new situation and environment. Rosen Work, Manual Lymphatic Drainage, Feldenkrais, The Trager Approach, Micro Movement, Cranial Sacral work, Orthobionomy, Jin Shin Jyutsu, Reflexology, Acupressure, and Esalen Massage are all types of bodywork that can be adapted to working with the aged and the ill. For the frail elderly and the seriously ill, even more subtle methods of touch may need to be employed.

Those who already have some knowledge of therapeutic massage will need to make certain adjustments in technique in order to administer massage to those in later life stages. The techniques that might be used in doing therapeutic massage or bodywork on a healthy and/or younger person are not always appropriate or desirable when working with those who are less active, aged, and/or seriously ill.

Individuals who are healthy and active can often tolerate one hour or longer of deep massage and full-body work. A Compassionate Touch session may be only fifteen to twenty minutes in duration. In general, the massage techniques used when working with those in later life stages are softer, gentler, and practiced for a shorter period of time than those that are used when administering therapeutic massage to younger and/or more physically active people.

There are many people who have never formally studied any particular form of bodywork or massage yet they instinctively know how to touch someone in a comforting and healing way. Many parents administer this kind of touch regularly to their children without even thinking about it. The ability to know when, where, and how to comfort their child through attentive touch grows out of their love for that child.

If you are interested in learning more about therapeutic massage, there are many how-to books on the market that include pictures, drawings, and clear instructions on how to practice a wide variety of bodywork techniques. If you are a beginning student in the art of massage therapy, you can learn a lot from reading such books. You can learn even more from taking some classes or workshops from an experienced teacher/trainer. You can learn best from your own direct experience and practice.

There are people for whom the word "massage" has negative connotations. It may conjure up visions of a body being kneaded into a bruised pulp, or it may be linked with something of an illicit or sexual nature. In addition, older people may think of massage as a self-indulgent activity for the hedonistic or the wealthy only.

If it seems to you that someone could benefit from attention in the form of touch and is hesitant to accept it, it might be because the person is uncomfortable with the word massage, or because he or she is unclear about what the word implies. If so, you can avoid using the word massage until the person understands from experience what you are actually offering. You can offer to put some lotion on the hands of a person who seems hesitant to let you touch him or her, or say you are giving back rubs to anyone who would like one today. You can assure the person no clothing need be removed and that he or she need not get out of bed. You may need to start out sitting beside such people, or asking if you might just hold a hand, until trust is established. Proceed slowly, and always with their permission, so that they do not feel overwhelmed.

If you sense that a person would be more comfortable, initially, with a loved one or caregiver staying in the room while you work with him or her, you might suggest that arrangement. It may reassure that person and reinforce the legitimacy of what you are doing. It may also help the caregiver or loved one to feel more comfortable about using touch as a part of caregiving.

I was once working with a cancer patient who was very close to death. The day I arrived for what turned out to be my last session with this person, the patient's sister asked if she could stay in the room and observe what I was doing. I was happy for her to do so, and after the patient died, I received a note from this woman telling me that being present for the Compassionate Touch session had given her the confidence to touch and stroke her loved one in the short time they had left together.

Sometimes the opposite phenomenon is true, and you will find it difficult to work with someone while that person's primary caregiver or close family member is nearby. The person you are touching may become confused or overwhelmed by the divided focus, may be conflicted about which person to relate to or may simply find it difficult to relax while the more familiar person is present. In such a case, you might gently suggest that the caregiver take a break and relax for a few minutes while you are working. If the caregiver sees that you are comfortable and confident about being alone with the person you are massaging, he or she will usually respond to such a suggestion.

The physical contact given in a Compassionate Touch session can range from attentively holding a person's hand, to a full body massage given to someone in a hospital bed instead of on a massage table. The particular skills and techniques employed by the massage practitioner may vary greatly from individual to individual and even with the same individual from one session to the next.

The types of therapeutic massage techniques used in Compassionate Touch can be divided into two major categories which often overlap: **sensitive massage** and **active holding**. Sensitive Massage would include pressure, squeezing or gentle kneading, moisturizing, and stroking. The category of active holding would include attentive (or conscious) touch, lifting/shifting, stretching/pulling and range of motion movements. Sensitive Massage also includes what might be called psychic touch, or "holding," the individual in your consciousness, maintaining contact with that person through all your senses, your physical presence, and your focused attention.

Sensitive Massage

People who are aging, ill, and/or approaching death have varying degrees of tolerance for and responsiveness to touch. It is necessary to proceed with sensitivity and caution when administering therapeutic massage to such individuals. It is much better to begin with a light and gentle touch and then gradually increase pressure (in whatever technique is being used) than to cause discomfort by using too much pressure to start with.

Pressure massage, combined with stroking, may be administered with the fingertips of both hands simultaneously almost anywhere on the body. The most common way to administer stronger pressure massage is probably with the thumbs. The entire upper back can be worked in this way, with the thumbs moving down the back simultaneously or in an alternating pattern, being careful never to press directly on the spine or on the scapula (shoulder blades).

Most often, pressure massage is combined with small, circular thumb movements in a pattern covering an area such as the shoulders or back but can also be used on the arch of the foot or on the palm of the hand. This technique may be used while working over clothing or directly on the skin.

Even quite elderly and fragile looking people can often take quite a bit of pressure on certain areas of the body such as the large trapezius muscles (which cross the tops of the shoulders) and the rhomboids (between the scapula and the spine). You can work on the rhomboid muscles with the thumbs by standing behind the back of a seated person. You might work on this same area with your fingertips by reaching underneath the shoulder and upper back while a person is lying face up in bed.

Pressure massage may also be used with lotion or oil, in which case the thumbs or fingertips would simply glide from one spot to the next without lifting off, and the pressure would be continuous. Pressure may be applied with the thumbs moving down the back either simultaneously or in an alternating pattern, on either side of the spine, with or without the use of oil.

Squeezing is usually accomplished with both hands simultaneously on extremities such as the legs or arms. This technique can best be described as opening and closing the hands around the body part being worked on. Squeezing, with either light or firm pressure, can be done over clothing or even coverings like blankets or quilts, and it can also be done directly on the skin.

Moisturizing is normally combined with stroking the skin in some way and is done for one of two reasons. You may apply lotion for the purpose of moisturizing and relieving dry skin. You might also apply lotion or oil as a skin lubricant to reduce friction while massaging. Types of lotions and oils for both purposes, as well as suitable containers for storing and using these lubricants, are discussed in Chapter Four.

In applying lotion or oil, squeeze a small amount into the palm of your hand and rub your hands together before touching a person's body. This will warm the oil or lotion (lotion takes longer to warm than oil), and it will warm your hands. Avoid pouring or squeezing any lubricant directly onto another person's

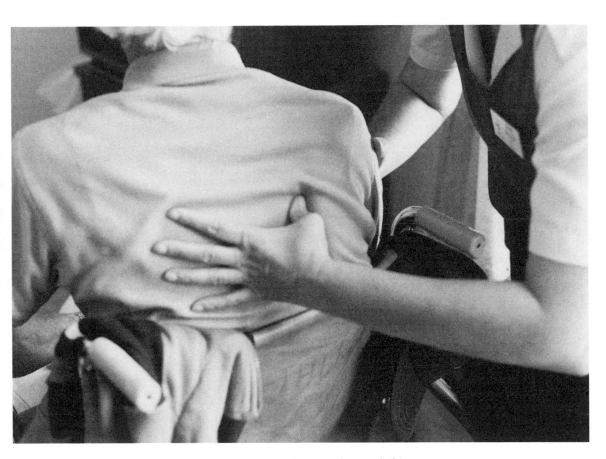

pressure massage using thumb over clothing

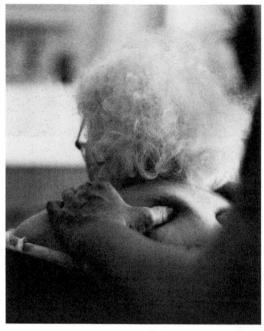

pressure massage with thumbs

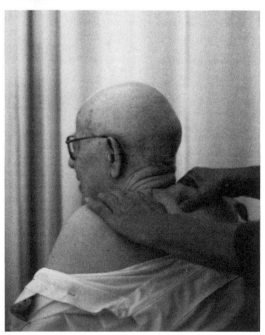

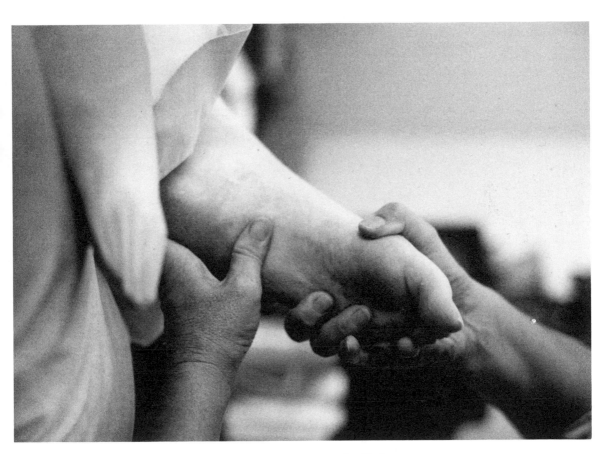

pressure massage on arch of foot

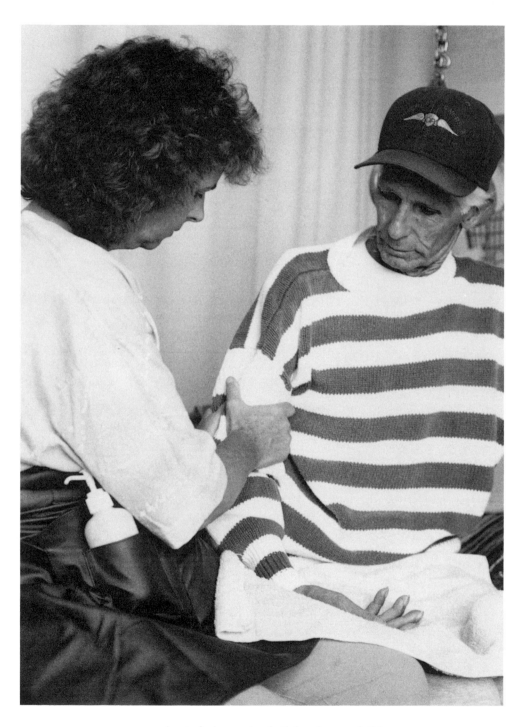

squeezing technique using both hands over clothing

body. Contacting the individual you are about to massage with your hands is more direct, more intimate, and more pleasurable.

A smooth, cool lotion may feel refreshing to a fevered body. Cold oil on skin is not usually a pleasant sensation however, so if your oil is at all cool, warm it as described above or as explained in Chapter Four. Use oil (or a combination of lotion and oil) primarily for long massage strokes on the arms, legs, or back. Keep the bottle close by (in an apron or massage belt, or set on a nearby table) so that you can easily get more lubricant as you need it. If you are using lotion, you can squeeze a bit of it onto your forearm so that you do not have to let go of someone's hand in order get more lubricant. Some skin absorbs moisture quite rapidly and other types of skin do not need a lot of extra lubrication. Use enough lubricant so that your hands can glide easily and smoothly up and down the area you are stroking. You can use lotion to moisturize dry hands or feet or even parts of the face. Moisturize another's hands or feet with lotion the same way you would your own, covering the entire area well, using the palms and fingers of both your hands. Make sure you pay attention to the areas between fingers and toes. You can make a natural transition from moisturizing to massaging if the person is open to continued touch.

As you moisturize a foot, for instance, you can begin to gently squeeze with both hands around the middle part of the foot or with one hand around the heel. You might apply a little pressure with short up and down or circular strokes with your fingertips or with your thumbs on the arch of the foot. You might then move on up the leg to the knees, applying oil or lotion on the upstroke and letting your hands wrap around the leg so that they slide down the back side of the leg, applying a bit of pressure to the calf muscles with your fingertips. When you reach the ankle, you can repeat this leg stroke, getting more oil or lotion as you need it, or you can continue down over the foot with one hand on top and one on the bottom.

Similarly, as you moisturize a hand, you can move up onto the forearm with short strokes and, if the person seems receptive, go ahead and gradually moisturize and massage the rest of the arm. Hold the person's wrist securely in one hand, let your other hand mold itself to the shape of the arm and slide smoothly all the way up the arm and onto the top of the shoulder circling around the shoulder and gliding down the back of the arm to the hand. You can then hold the wrist with your right hand and let your left hand glide up the inside of the arm and back down.

If the person you are working with is in a hospital or home bed, you can position your chair at the side of the bed or possibly sit or stand at the end of the bed to work on the feet and legs. If the bed is on rollers and can be easily moved, you can stand at the other end to work on the head, face, neck, and shoulders.

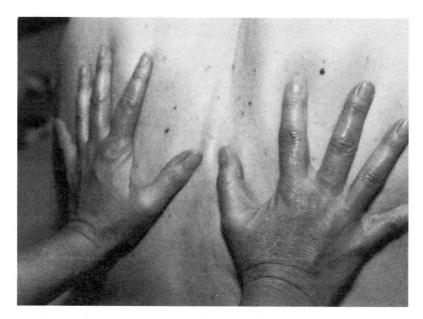

pressure massage \ stroking with oil

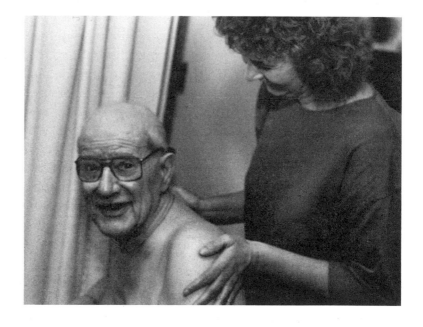

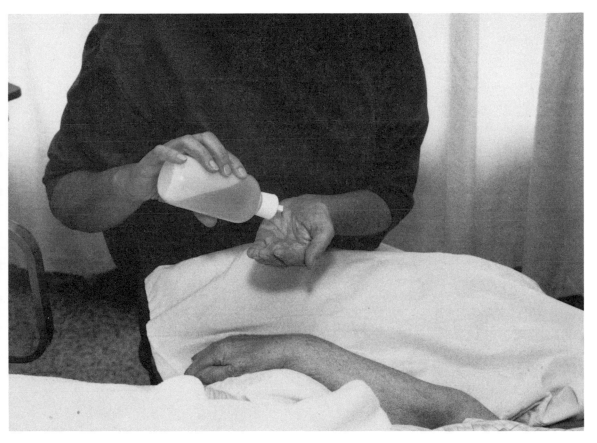

pouring lubricant into palm of hand

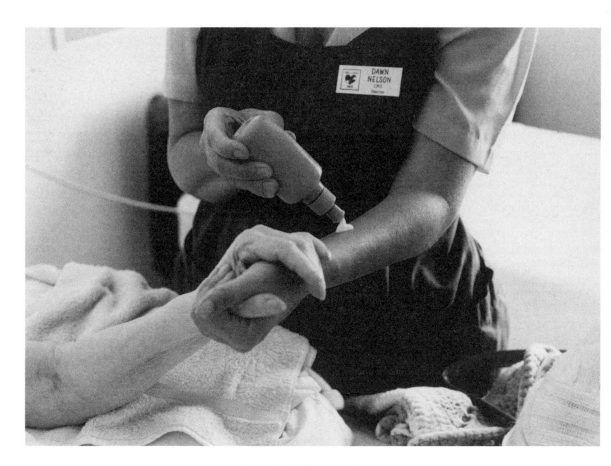

squeezing lotion onto forearm

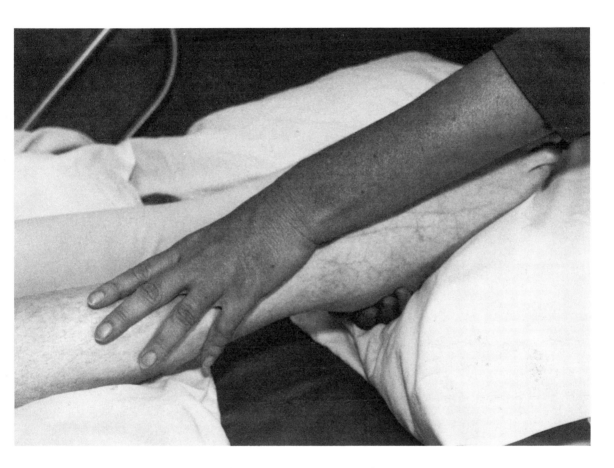

holding ankle secure while moisturing \ stroking

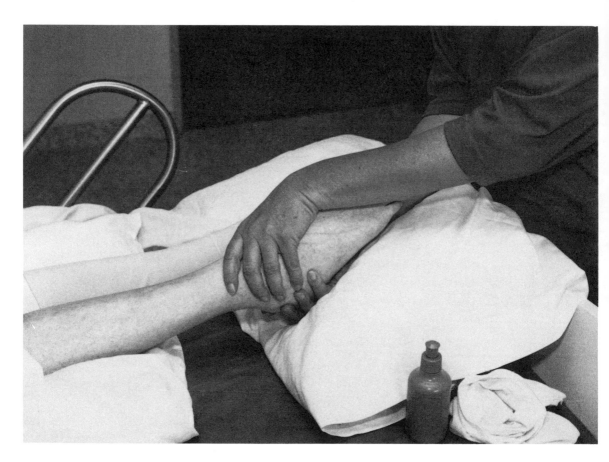

continuation of moisturizing \ stroking onto foot

gentle squeezing/pressure combined with moisturizing back of leg

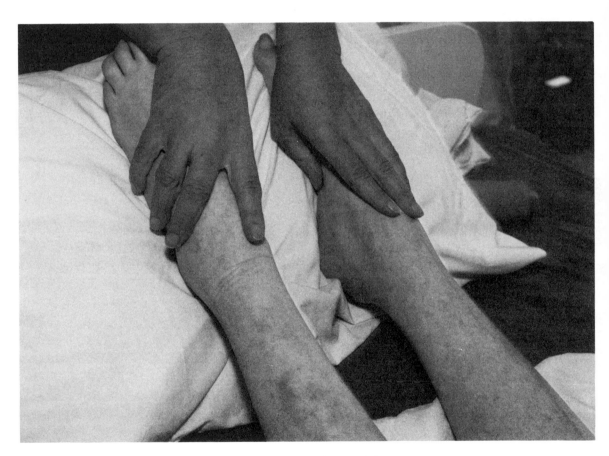

moisturizing \ stroking both feet

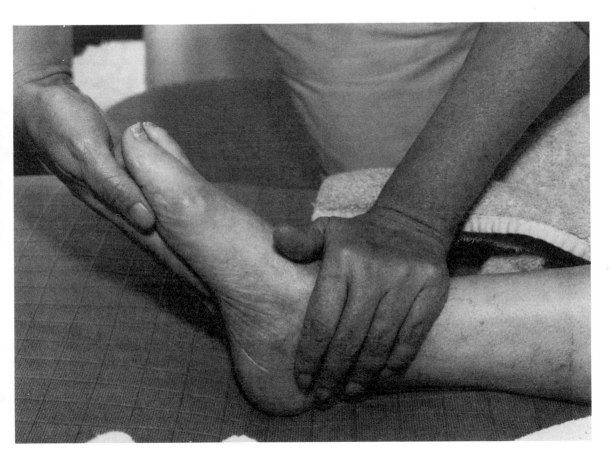

working one foot at a time

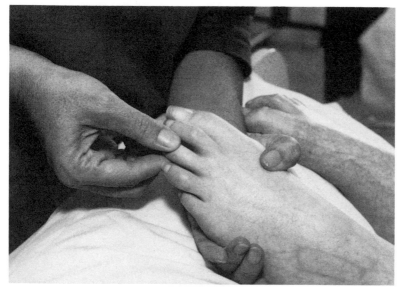

working each toe

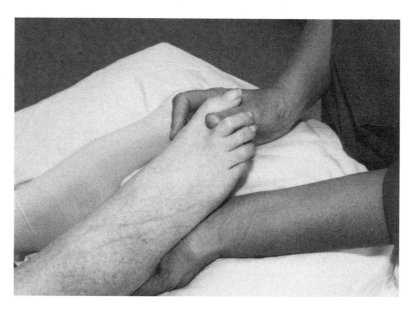

working between toes

Remember that you can raise or lower hospital beds! This gives you more options and allows you to work more comfortably. If a height adjustment is not possible or you sense that such movement (and the accompanying sound) would be too jarring to a patient, then you must adjust your own height by placing blankets or pillows on your chair, possibly sitting on the bed with the person, getting down on your knees on the floor, or doing whatever works!

Whatever techniques you are using, always work on both sides of the body so that you leave the person with a sense of balance and completeness in terms of your attention and in terms of the physical stimulation and body awareness that your touch initiates. This principle applies even if the person has no feeling in one side of the body. If a leg or arm is missing, be sure to massage whatever part is still there.

One lady I have worked with for about six months has, among other problems, only partial use of her right arm due to a stroke. In the beginning she wanted me to spend our whole session together just massaging her "bad" arm, although I always offered to do a little work on her other extremities. I eventually discovered that she was holding on to a belief that massage therapy alone would bring back the feeling in her arm. She frequently complained that I didn't come often enough and never spent enough time with her (thinking, I came to realize, that the more time I spent massaging her arm, the quicker her body would be back to "normal"). She told me she was relying on me completely and was not going to physical therapy (which may or may not have actually been the case).

One day I offered to spend a little extra time with this lady and persuaded her to let me massage her other arm and her legs. I acknowledged the frustration she must be feeling about the loss of control over her physical body. I let her know that massage alone could not "heal" her paralysis and told her some of the benefits our sessions could provide, with her participation. I noticed that she seemed more relaxed and more willing to let me move on to work with others after I had done some massage on both sides of her body, acknowledged the reality of her situation, and was honest about what our time together might and might not accomplish. I hope this lady and I can continue to work together in helping her achieve acceptance and balance in her physical/mental state as it exists so that a way may be opened in which her therapy can progress.

Active Holding

A cancer patient whom I had been seeing for some weeks gradually lost feeling in most of her body. I continued to moisturize her skin and to do deeper massage on one arm and hand where she still had sensation. One day, at a loss as to what I could do that might be helpful to her, I stopped moving my hands and simply let them come to rest on her arm. As I sat beside her, remaining in physical contact and experiencing our connection, she surprised me by asking "What are you doing when you move around and then stop like that?" Since I had not been trying to "do" anything, I replied that I was simply remaining "in touch" with her. She responded, "Well, it's very calming." This was a good reminder that people do experience a difference between conscious physical contact and casual, random touch.

There will be times when the most compassionate thing you can do for another, in contacting that person on a physical level, is what might be called **attentive touch.** A person's body may simply be too sensitive or too traumatized to take any more pressure or movement than the gentlest of touches or movement. Sometimes a person who is near death is becoming de-identified with the body, and it simply becomes inappropriate to do anything other than hold a hand or make some other kind of gentle but conscious physical contact. It may be the lightest touch with a fingertip or two at the top of the head or the bottom of the feet; it may be your hand on top of the bed covers softly molded around a wrist or ankle. The point is to be conscious of the physical connection as you make it. As you actively and attentively make the contact, you must focus your awareness not just on the person's physical body, but on the individual whose body you are touching. Keep in mind that you are contacting the individual through the physical act of touch. Taking a person's hand between both of yours as you hold that individual in your consciousness is an appropriate, reassuring, and soothing form of contact. It is one good way to begin a Compassionate Touch session. You can sense a great deal about a person's physical condition by holding his or her hand. You will be able to tell something about the person's strength and energy by the way in which that person returns (or does not return) your touch. The temperature of the skin can give you an indication of how well the blood is circulating and about how active he or she may be. You can pick up information about the individual, with this initial touch, that will help you in deciding how to proceed in the session.

Actively holding one or both hands of the person you have been working with is also one way to end a Compassionate Touch session. If you start the session with the hands, coming back to a similar simple touch after touching or massaging other parts of the body can bring a sense of completion and balance to your interaction with that individual in that particular session. If your interaction has been verbal as well as physical, then sitting in silence for a few moments with your hands entwined can be calming and restful to both of you.

There are also times when holding someone's hand between both of yours for an extended period of time may comprise the whole session. The individual you are contacting will benefit from your active physical connection as well as from your attention and your presence. The tender loving touch of the human hand can be a powerful nonverbal form of communication. There are times when that touch alone is much more effective than any words one could say.

The first patient I was given as a new Hospice volunteer was a woman whose body was riddled with cancer. I had been told that she would most likely be alive only a few more days. Her skin was pale but translucent and her eyes were large and beautiful in her thin face. She was weak and did not talk much though she indicated that she enjoyed the gentle foot massage I gave her. I also moisturized her arms and hands with lotion. When I went back a couple of days later and asked if she'd like a foot massage, she said in a barely audible voice, "let's just skip that today shall we?" So I sat in a chair beside her bed while her husband went out to pick up a few groceries. I took one of her hands between both of mine and the two of us stayed together in this sacred silence for nearly 20 minutes. I kept my attention on her when her eyes were closed, and when they flickered open, I simply met her gaze and continued holding her hand, conscious of our physical contact and aware of a deeper connection that was taking place.

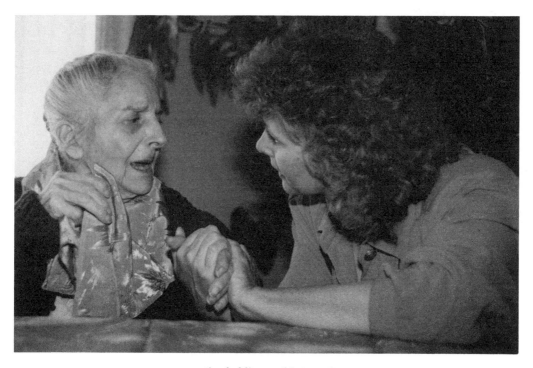

active holding and interaction

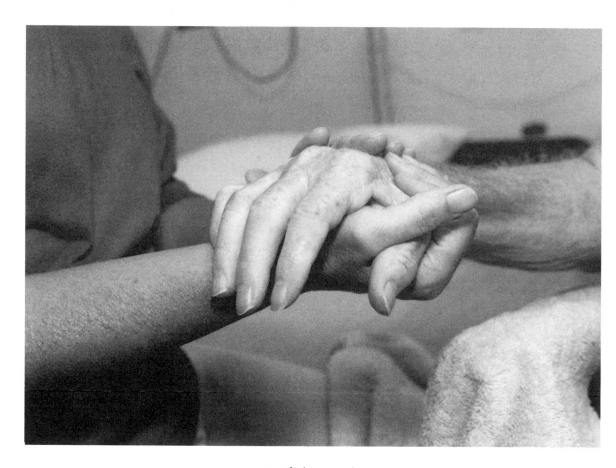

completing a session

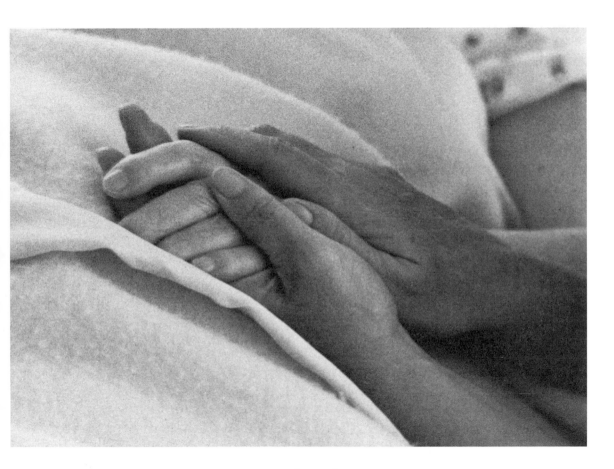

attentive touch

Even those who find a great deal of pleasure in being massaged and stroked may be unable to enjoy such contact as their illness progresses and changes occur in their physical and mental state. You will need to adjust your touch accordingly and remain physically present with the individual in a way that is comforting and supportive. You can try placing one hand on top of a person's head with the other over the heart, or gently cupping the head with a hand on either side, or perhaps actively holding one of the person's hands while your other hand rests on his or her belly or chest.

There may come a time when even the most sensitive massage is too much or when even the gentlest touch becomes almost intolerable to someone you have been working with. If any kind of physical contact is uncomfortable, you can still maintain what I would call **psychic touch** with your loved one, patient, or client. In other words, you stay mentally connected to the individual and in close physical proximity, with all your senses attentive to both the body and the being you are with. The person will experience your physical and mental presence on some level. Your conscious attention can give that person comfort and support so that he or she feels less isolated and alone.

You can effectively use attentive touch on other parts of the body, such as the shoulders. For example, you might stand behind a person confined to a wheelchair and gently place both of your hands on the tops of the shoulders, letting your fingers rest naturally over the front of the shoulders. In this case, you are not pressing down on the shoulders in any way. You are simply resting your hands on the body in a conscious and attentive way.

As you use this or other attentive touch techniques, be aware of the energy flowing out through your hands. Stay present with the individual whose body you are touching and stay awake to the energetic contact your touch creates. You can remain in this kind of contact for as long as you wish. When it seems appropriate, break the contact by allowing your hands to rise slowly up and away from the person's body. Allow a few moments for the effect of this contact to be absorbed before continuing with the same technique or some other one. You might also use this touch on top of the shoulders as the initial contact for a neck, shoulder, and upper back massage.

I recall placing my hands on the shoulders of a ninety-seven-year-old nursing home patient as she sat in her wheelchair. I came to know this woman as a dear old lady, usually quite alert and talkative though a little hard of hearing. At the time I first met her, she had never had any kind of massage in her life but seemed open to a new experience. As I stood behind her wheelchair and brought my hands into contact with her body, I felt her shoulders drop and experienced her whole body relax as a result of this simple contact. Later in that first session, this lady took an almost childlike delight in having her hands and fingers massaged.

She enjoyed being touched so much that we continued our sessions together until she died peacefully in her ninety-eighth year of life.

The pressure you use with attentive touch can range from the very lightest contact to a fairly firm holding or enclosing. It depends on the condition of the person whom you are touching, what you intuitively feel is appropriate, and the feedback you are receiving. If you are unsure of how much pressure to use and the person is able to respond either verbally or in some other manner, you can ask a direct question, "Is this too much for you?" or "Would you like more pressure here?"

If you have ever been struck by a flu virus, you may recall what it feels like to be bedridden with a fevered, aching, and weakened body. Sometimes it even seems as if moving to a different position on the bed might take more energy than you have available. Imagine being in this state for weeks or months! Massage can provide welcome relief to muscles that ache from disuse and disease, yet sometimes the movement of some therapeutic massage techniques can feel like too much stimulation. In such cases, something as seemingly simple as just lifting a leg and shifting it to a new position may be experienced by the person inhabiting that weakened body as merciful attention.

When lifting any body limb, be sure that you give adequate attention and support to this movement so that the person feels secure. In the case of a leg, put one hand under the heel or around the middle part of the foot and the other hand around the calf. Lift the leg a few inches and perhaps suspend it in air for a moment before gently lowering it back down onto the bed just an inch or two to the right or left of the previous spot.

Elevating the leg slightly by placing a small pillow under the heel of a foot or rolled up towel under an ankle may help provide a needed shift in position for a bedridden patient who is too weak to move herself. A bed pillow under the knees for awhile may help circulation and relieve strain on lower back muscles. Gently bending a straightened arm and placing a person's hand over the heart or belly area can provide a needed positional shift and may also feel comforting. Raising the head slightly and putting a small roll pillow under the neck, or just lifting and holding the head while you fluff up the bed pillow, gently replacing the head on the pillow, provides a weakened person with a moment of attentive touch and moves the neck muscles so that they don't become "frozen."

You can "lift" a shoulder of a patient on his or her back by carefully raising the shoulder off the bed as far as is comfortable for the patient and letting it rest again in its natural position. This movement can be gently and slowly repeated several times on each shoulder. While the shoulder is lifted, you can reach under the upper back in order to do some circular stroking or fingertip pressure. If you are working directly on the skin, you can achieve a nice stroke on the back by moisturizing one hand with a bit of oil or lotion, placing it under the upper back as you lift a shoulder, leaving it there after the shoulder is let down and then slowly pulling the hand out.

Any body extremity that can tolerate such movement may be lifted off its resting place for a few moments in repeated sequences, giving the skin a rest, increasing body awareness, and stimulating circulation. Gently stretching or slightly pulling on an arm or leg can sometimes feel good, and this technique is easily combined with lifting and/or shifting.

Range of motion exercises can be incorporated into a Compassionate Touch session as an alternative or additional technique. This technique can be used in working with individuals in regaining or increasing control of limbs after a stroke, for instance, or in regaining movement following an injury or a long illness.

Focusing attention on specific parts of the body increases body awareness in general. When people are too weak to move their own bodies, moving the limbs for them provides a form of mild exercise, which can improve circulation and stimulate the brain. In a manner of speaking, the movement is like "oiling the joints" in the body so that they don't get rusty. In helping people to increase the range of motion available to them in the use of body extremities such as arms or legs, it is advisable to start very slowly and gradually increase the movement. If people are able to initiate movement on their own encourage them to do so. This will give them a sense of control, progress, and accomplishment, while increasing their body awareness.

Range of motion may be explored through circular, linear, or lateral movements, in most cases, wherever a body part is connected to another body part by joints—fingers, wrists, forearms, ankles, arms, and legs. For a person who has remained inactive and/or immobile over a longer period of time, working to increase range of movement will be gradual and sometimes very subtle. It is important to give positive feedback and encouragement.

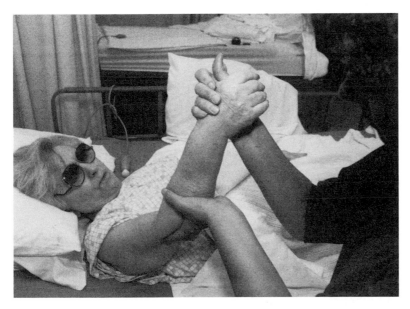

lifting \ shifting and range of motion

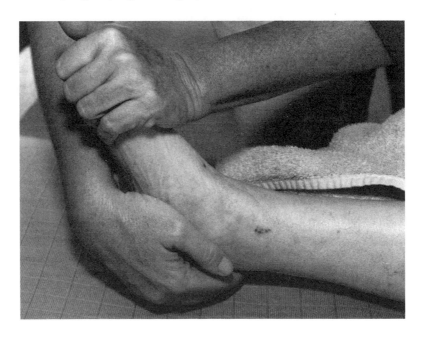

Listening/Feedback Skills

Listening is often a crucial component in a Compassionate Touch session. People who are in crisis as well as those who feel isolated, alone, or abandoned need to talk and are grateful for someone who takes the time to listen!

Active listening is a communication skill that becomes a highly valued art when practiced consciously. An active listener will:

- stay awake
- be alert and present in the moment
- remain open to the other individual
- be interested in receiving the communication presented
- understand as well as he or she can
- not evaluate or judge what is presented
- resist interruptions and distractions
- ask for clarification so that misunderstanding does not escalate
- acknowledge that a communication has been received

The ability to truly listen without interrupting or commenting, the ability to actually receive what others are trying to communicate, is, in and of itself, a significant and powerful technique.

Reflective feedback is a kind of communication that can arise out of active listening. It is communication that reflects or mirrors back to the one who has been talking, what you, as the listener, actually heard and understood. The point is not to repeat the exact words that were spoken but to test your understanding of what was said by reflecting back to the communicator in your own words what you heard. Reflective feedback is an excellent way to avoid some of the misunderstandings and problems that arise in relating to others.

Interpretive feedback goes a step further than reflective feedback in that you, as the listener, interpret what the person has said before reflecting it back to them. For instance a person may be complaining in a loud voice about his or her care in some way—"The food is never hot;" "They always keep me waiting;" "They make me take a bath..." You might respond to the last outburst by saying, "You don't want to take a bath," or you might say, "It must be difficult to have so little control over your life." One response is reflective and the other one is interpretive. The first response is an acknowledgement in the sense that you have received and understood what the person is communicating. The second response is an acknowledgement of something deeper that the person is trying to get across, of what that person may be experiencing underneath the words that have been spoken. By your interpretive feedback, you are actually giving that individual an opening to access and express his or her deeper feelings.

On more than one occasion, when I've been working with the "terminally" ill, a person has asked me if I could give him or her something to hasten death. Rather than begin a discussion on the philosophical, moral, or legal implications of such a request, I have tried to acknowledge not just the words but the feelings beneath the words which I heard. In one case, I responded by asking, "Are you feeling that you are ready to die now?" This is another example of interpretive feedback.

In any case, avoid evaluating, judging, or commenting on what your loved one or someone with whom you are working may say. Be careful, also, about continually sharing your own experiences. Self-disclosure may occasionally be supportive and appropriate, but your own experience should be shared only if it would be truly helpful to the person you are serving. It is usually best to simply listen, with all your available senses, understand as well as you can, and receive what the person is communicating. You can check out your understanding through either reflective or interpretive feedback when possible. When you understand what the other person is trying to get across, acknowledge that fact by saying something such as "Thank you," or "I understand," or "I get it." Remember that you do not have to agree with what someone says in order to acknowledge receiving the thought! This experience of completing communication cycles is, unfortunately, absent in life to a large degree. When real communication actually takes place, it is not only satisfying, it is empowering and healing in the deepest sense.

Visualization and Guided Fantasy

Creative visualization, forming pictures or images in the mind's eye, works quite well as both an affirmation and a relaxation technique for some people. Guiding or directing someone else in creating images in the mind is a technique that has been widely and successfully used as an aid in pain control and stress management, for fostering self-awareness, and as a psychological tool or process leading to deeper insight and clarity. The number of commercially produced cassette tapes now on the market that contain guided fantasies and visualization exercises attests to the popularity and accessibility of this modality. I know many people who use such tapes as a sleep inducing aid, as a help in pain and stress control, and/or to achieve deep states of peace and relaxation. The success of this type of technique is a powerful indicator of how thoughts can influence both physical and emotional states.

The dimension of touch, along with the voice of a real and accessible person, can escalate the benefits of a guided visualization technique. You may assist an individual through the use of guided visualization, for instance, in becoming aware of his or her breath and breathing patterns. You may be able to help someone move from shallow chest breathing to a deeper and more relaxing abdominal or belly breathing. You can direct a person's attention to specific parts of the body as you are touching or massaging that part by giving a verbal instruction to the person to bring his or her attention to that place.

If you are working with an ill or an aged person who is mentally alert enough to follow your directions, you might ask that person to visualize "untying" a knotted muscle as you gently massage it. Or, you could tell the person to imagine that the breath is a particular color and then direct the person to "send" his or her breath into the tense area. You might try asking someone to imagine the tension or tightness as a hard block of ice that then dissolves or becomes liquid, or a rope with many knots that turns into a ribbon of smoke. You can make up any image that you sense might work for a particular individual. When you find the right image, the results can be almost magical. Be sure to point out to people you work with in this manner that they can use this technique on their own, without you. Never abuse others by making them think that you are the one "doing" the relaxing or creating the change in state that they experience.

You might use guided fantasy as a stress-reducing or calming device by helping a person to create a tranquil and beautiful scene of some kind in the mind's eye, a peaceful space/place where that person feels comfortable, safe, and happy. If you are able to ascertain, through asking questions or through written records, something about a person's life before his or her incapacitation, you may be able to find something to use as a jumping off place in creating such a fantasy. If someone was an expert mountain climber, for instance, you could start with that image. If you know that someone with whom you are working enjoyed vacationing in Hawaii every year, you might begin by asking that person to imagine her or himself walking along a seashore, feeling the warm sun beaming down and the sand underfoot. You could then go on to guide that person in mentally creating an idyllic island scene. Be sure to have the person you are guiding visualize him or herself in the scene. Encourage the person to add to the scene everything he or she would desire to make the place or the situation perfect in every way—favorite foods, flowers, weather, other people, animal companions, and so on.

Most people are eventually able to visualize their "special place" without a voice guiding them. They will be able to mentally create their ideal scene any time they choose to, and to experience themselves relaxing into the peaceful, contented state that the scene evokes.

In the case of the alert aged, you might use a visualization technique as both a relaxation process, to elicit personal remembrances, or as an aid in creating oral histories. I have observed quite elderly and frail people take on youthful characteristics as they relive important events in their lives by talking about them to someone who cares enough to listen. Their eyes start to sparkle, color comes to the skin, and they become animated and cheerful as they are encouraged to expand on happy memories, talk about career accomplishments, or share some special experience.

One lady I used to visit in a long-term care facility was always very quiet as I moisturized and massaged her extremities until one day she made a comment about how boring her life was. I asked her what kinds of things she used to like to do and her whole countenance changed as she immediately responded, "Dancing!" I began to ask her questions about what kind of dancing, who she went dancing with, what her favorite music was, and so on until she had painted a "moving" picture for me of her nights out on the town in San Francisco with her girlfriends. I looked forward to expanding this scene with her each time we were together for not only did they give me a much fuller understanding of this woman's life, but she found pleasure in recreating and sharing those memories with me.

You might ask a person to close his or her eyes and concentrate on the inhalation and exhalation of the breath as you administer a foot massage. After the person begins to relax, ask him or her to remember a particularly happy or significant event (when the person felt the strongest or most proud, for example). You can guide and encourage someone in recreating a scene and then help that person expand the scene to include sense memory by asking specific questions about the time of year, the weather, colors, sights, sounds, and so on. You are working on improving a person's circulation on the physical level, through massage, while that person is improving his or her mental and emotional circulation, so to speak, through this type of visualization and sense memory process.

Guided Meditation and Exploration

Meditation is a means of directing thought or focusing attention, of bringing conscious awareness to each moment as it arises. The practice itself could be something as simple as keeping one's attention concentrated on one's own breathing, focusing on the flame of a candle as it burns, or the conscious repetition of a meaningful word or sound. Anything can be used as a vehicle for sensitizing and focusing the mind in moment- to-moment awareness.

Guided meditations, which use spoken words as a focus for the mind, can be used in conjunction with administering therapeutic massage or touch. Such work is especially helpful if you are working with someone who is experiencing pain—physical, emotional, and/or mental—and who is interested in meeting that pain with mercy, nonjudgement, and love instead of with denial or fear.

We often try to lessen the sensations and emotions we label "pain" by pretending they don't exist, by ignoring them, or by distracting ourselves in any and every way we can think of. Such resistance seems to increase rather than decrease our suffering. Often, simply putting our attention on our discomfort (sorrow, anguish, fear ...) and acknowledging its existence can reduce it drastically. Describing our experience, communicating it to someone else, is also a way of acknowledging and alleviating pain.

You may support someone in bringing discomfort into conscious awareness through words as well as through your real contact with that person. If the person you are working with is able to communicate verbally, you might ask him or her to describe the pain to you. Where is it located? How big is it? What color is it? Does the pain have a shape? Is it round, flat, rough, smooth, hot, cold? If you are working with people who are not verbal, simply ask them to notice these things.

As you observe, on a physical level, holding patterns in one's body (muscles contracted around an incision, injury, or wound, for instance), ask that person to notice what thoughts arise in regard to the discomfort, or what feelings he or she might experience while holding the attention on that part of the body. The person may do this silently or may share his or her thoughts and feelings with you as you continue to guide this meditative exploration. You might ask a person to breathe into the pain, surround the pain with love, or to touch the pain with forgiveness. This kind of exercise in awareness can help an individual to detach or de-identify from intense emotional states. It can change the relationship of the individual to the pain that is being experienced, thus reducing anxiety and suffering.

Never force any technique or process on someone who is not open to receiving it or who is not at least willing to try it. If you insist on using a technique with someone who is resistant to you or to the technique, not only will the potential benefits of the technique go unrealized but the relationship between you and that individual will be damaged.

Shared Breathing

Bringing your breath into harmony with the breathing pattern of the person you are touching can give an even deeper dimension to your connection with that individual. You can use this technique at any time while you are working with someone and it may sometimes even happen spontaneously. As a practice, the technique of shared breathing involves becoming conscious first of your own breathing as you inhale and exhale. It next requires putting your attention on the breathing pattern of the other person. You can then begin to adjust the rhythm of your own breathing in order to synchronize your inhalation and exhalation of breath with the other person's. When practiced at length, shared breathing can evolve into a surprisingly powerful exercise. It often creates a sense of peace in both participants. It can heighten awareness of the breathing process and of the relationship or connection between two individuals. It may even produce a deep emotional catharsis in one or both people.

When someone is quite ill and/or near death, that person's breathing may become irregular, in which case it becomes more difficult, though not impossible, to synchronize your breathing. You may be able to help such a person breathe into each moment as it unfolds (much as you would support a woman in natural childbirth) by staying in contact with the individual and perhaps talking that person through each breath.

I was recently sitting with a man whom I'd become quite fond of in the relatively short time we had spent together. The illness he had fought for two years had wasted his body. He had eventually become too weak to move or even speak, yet the light in his eyes was still bright and he continued to smile sweetly at me from time to time. He could also muster the strength to squeeze my hand occasionally and no other communication seemed necessary. The predominant sound and movement in those intimate moments was the breath moving in and out of this man's frail body. After awhile, I noticed that my friend was holding his breath frequently, perhaps in resistance to some physical discomfort or in resistance to the experience of dying. I began to encourage him, both verbally and with gentle touch over his chest, to let his breath flow in and out rather than holding it. I thanked him each time he complied with the instruction. Every time I noticed him holding his breath, I would whisper again, "let the breath go," as I rested a hand on his chest or moved my hand ever so gently back and forth on his belly. He looked at me questioningly at one point and I said softly, "You're holding your breath." "Oh," he responded, smiling as if amused by the joke. Then he exhaled and we continued breathing together in silence.

As emphasized earlier, Compassionate Touch is not a set of prescribed techniques to be followed, but merciful and *care*-full service that unfolds in the reality of relationship. The Compassionate Touch practitioner must employ both natural abilities and learned skills in working with each individual and must then trust that new and appropriate ways of touch and supportive care will present themselves in the moment, as they are needed.

Communicating with the Dying

As people who are approaching death become weaker and begin to detach or de-identify with their physical existence, they may begin to communicate in more symbolic language, in regressed language, or without the use of words. It is important to stay open to receiving the communication that is offered, in whatever form it may take.

When an individual who is near death speaks of not being at home or wondering where home is, for instance, caregivers may assume the person is confused from medication he or she may be taking, or that the disease from which the person suffers has affected the brain. The caregiver then becomes anxious and upset over the dying person's loss of ability to communicate. Some diseases do cause dementia as they progress, yet it is also common for a person nearing death to speak of home or wanting to go home as a way of indicating a desire to leave the body. A person may talk about needing a passport or a plane ticket, or wanting to get to the bus stop to communicate that he or she is ready to make a change or to go on to a new and different place. I remember my father talking about trying to get to the end of the football field shortly before he died. He told me once that he could see the lights on the other side of the field, but that he just couldn't seem to get to them. Caregivers can support the person making the transition and can share that individual's journey as long as possible by accepting, rather than refuting or denying, what is being said, and by letting the person know that whatever he or she wants is okay.

I remember a woman in the advanced stages of cancer who kept asking her husband to please close the door, pointing to a nearby wall. Her husband ignored the request at first and then told his wife that there was no open door where she was pointing. Finally, at her insistence, he walked over to the wall and went through the actions of shutting a door. I felt that perhaps this patient was simply trying to communicate that she wasn't ready to die. My hunch was confirmed when she turned to me after her husband left the room and said, "I'm not ready to go through the door yet." I assured her that when she was ready, the door would open for her again.

I have observed people who know they are nearing death regress in their use of language and begin using words that they used when first learning to speak. This may be especially true in the case of an adult child being cared for by a parent. I recently made a phone call to schedule my weekly session with a bedridden hospice patient in her early forties. Her mother, who had been caring for her night and day for some months, told me tearfully that she thought her daughter was "slipping away" from her. When I arrived at their home, the daughter was very weak but coherent, and she seemed to be intently focused on dying. I encouraged her mother to sit where she could maintain eye contact, as well as physical contact, with her daughter while I stayed on the other side of the bed, where I could stroke her back, administer gentle touch, and give support from behind. Time seemed to suspend in a sacred space as I witnessed these two women say good-bye to each other. The mother, with tears streaming down her face, told her daughter that she was releasing her, that she should just leave her body and float toward the light. The daughter told her mother how much she loved her and that she would miss her. After awhile, she began speaking in shortened phrases and a child-like voice. She would drift off and then open her eyes again, find her mother's face, and repeat, "I go bye-bye now . . . I go bye-bye." This continued throughout the day until she fell into a coma.

It is also possible that all speech will stop, yet the individual who is close to death will still communicate with those nearby through gestures and/or facial expressions. Sometimes a person will smile and reach out or seem to be visually focused on something or someone that no one else can see. Research has proved that in the near-death state, people often see loved ones who have already died, angels, lights, or other indescribably beautiful visions. Rather than feel excluded when someone nearing death seems to be aware of something that we are not aware of, we can share in the experience by staying consciously present and in contact with the person, accepting whatever seems to be happening for him or her.

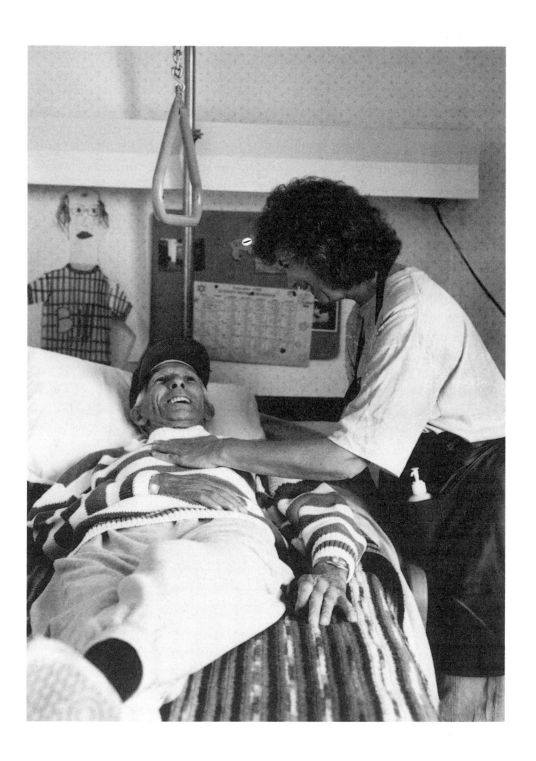

❦ 6 ❦

Guidelines And Suggestions

. . . can a society legitimately call itself civilized if it does not provide sensitive and human care to the elderly during the last days of their lives?

Jeanie Schmit Kayser-Jones

Before the Session

Do not practice Compassionate Touch with anyone if you are ill yourself! If you have a fever, flu, cold, or any possibility of a contagious disease, refrain from getting close to or touching a person who is already physically weak and vulnerable. For the frail and infirm, catching the flu could be very serious or even fatal.

It is also not a good idea to practice Compassionate Touch if you are extremely fatigued or in an emotional crisis. Unless you are able to override your own state of mind by focusing your attention on the other person, it will be felt on some level by the person receiving your touch. It will influence the session and could affect that individual adversely. Do your best to maintain your own physical and emotional health so that you will be able to administer massage or attentive touch when it is needed or requested.

When working with those in later life stages, it is wise to call a few hours before a scheduled appointment to confirm that you are coming. There may have been some significant change in the person's condition, including death, that would be important for you to know. An overwhelmed caregiver may have forgotten the appointment or gotten confused as to who was coming when. The patient may have been moved to a different place and no one remembered to get in touch with you. It is also important to inform those involved as soon as possible if you are unable to keep a scheduled appointment for any reason. Try to avoid any last minute disappointments for your clients/patients and/or caregivers.

Avoid wearing heavily scented perfumes or lotions to Compassionate Touch sessions. Dress simply and comfortably in clothing that will not hamper your work or be a distraction. File your fingernails short enough so that they will not interfere with fingertip massage techniques that you may be using. Leave bracelets and rings at home or remove them and put them in a safe place before you begin your hands-on caregiving session.

Before entering the home or the room of the person you will be touching, take a few moments to ground and center yourself. You don't have to do anything elaborate or visually weird in front of other people. You may want to meditate in your own home or a separate room before going to a session. You may choose to sit quietly in your car for a few moments before going into someone's home, or to pause briefly outside the door of a hospital room before entering. Put your attention on your own physicality and become aware of your connection to the ground beneath you.

Shifting your awareness to your breath, without even doing anything to change it, is a powerful focusing device. It can be quite effective as a calming and centering technique. Once your attention is focused on your breath, find the place in your body that you experience as your center and breathe deeply from that place.

I remember hesitating outside the home of the first hospice patient to whom I was assigned as a volunteer and the thought/prayer that arose in my mind was, "Please let me keep my heart open and my mouth shut." Sometimes, before approaching the person with whom I will be working, I repeat a silent meditative thought or affirmation; sometimes I just focus on my breathing for a few minutes, or I put my attention on opening my heart to include whatever it is that I may be fearful of or not wanting to accept in regard to a particular situation or individual.

It is my experience that it is best to let go of any notions one may have of "doing the right thing" and even of "helping." Approaching an individual with the attitude that we have the training or the skills or the right answers only gets in the way of real relationship.

Something else you may want to do before administering therapeutic touch is to energize your hands. There are many ways to do this. One way is to shake your hands vigorously to free them of tension and then rub the palms of your hands together rapidly a few times, generating heat and energy. Another way is to squeeze your hands into fists and then flick the fingers and thumbs outward, spreading the fingers apart and opening the hands until you feel the skin on your palms "stretching." You will feel a warm and tingly sensation in your hands after repeating this action a few times. You might visualize a stream of warm light radiating out from your heart, down through your arms, and into the palms of both hands. You can also try "breathing" into your hands by mentally following your breath as you exhale, directing it down your arms, into your hands, and out through your fingertips.

Let go of any preconceived ideas you may have about the person you are about to touch. Set aside your opinions about his or her particular situation or condition. Take lightly any evaluative comments made by others concerning someone's personality or way of being. You may be told that a person you are about to see is always angry or uncooperative, or that a patient is in "heavy denial." However, your experience with that particular individual may be quite different from someone else's. This has happened to me on several occasions. It is not necessary to invalidate your own experience or another person's perceptions, or to argue about the situation. If, however, you relate to people according to someone else's experience of their personality, or as if a written report about their condition is who they are, then your relationships with those people will lack reality in the present moment. Continue to approach each individual with an open mind and an open heart, each time that you come together.

Being open means being willing to have things be however they are. Make a conscious decision to remain open during the time you spend with others and to face whatever may occur. This will not always be an easy task. There may be times you will want to run away, give up, or give way to your own emotional reactions. These are natural impulses. Noticing your impulse and choosing to stay in contact with the person with whom you are working could have a significant effect on both of you.

This is not to say that you should never cry or let yourself be affected by what those you are working with may be experiencing. You have a responsibility to be real and you should take the risk to be real even if that means letting your sadness show. Avoid dramatizing, however, or going into your own emotional reaction to the point where a patient feels he or she must comfort you. Notice what is coming up for you, *and* avoid getting attached to your own emotions or shifting the attention to yourself. Keep your attention focused on the individual with whom you are working.

People suffering from dementia, such as Alzheimer's Disease and other kinds of age-related imbalances, are likely to forget who you are from visit to visit. They may confuse you with someone else, they may even become inexplicably hostile and lash out at you in some way. It is possible to handle irrational outbursts and radical mood swings by simply ignoring the behavior and remaining focused on the individual who happens to be behaving in that way. If someone you are working with should suddenly become aggressively angry and/or out of control, do not take it personally and do not allow yourself to be abused. Ask for help if you need it. Leave the room if you have to.

Before going in to begin a therapeutic massage session it is usually helpful to find out as much as you can from the nurse on duty, or from the caregiver or family member in charge regarding the physical condition of the person you are about to see. Ask about recent changes or if there is anything you need to know. It would be helpful to be informed, for instance, if a patient is receiving a medication that is known to produce significant side effects such as headaches, nausea, itching, insomnia, depression, mood swings, and so on. It is important for you to know if a person can stand or walk alone, and how much assistance he or she may need in turning in bed or in getting from one place to another. Remember, mental and emotional states can greatly affect physical conditions and vice versa. Remember, too, that whatever condition or state a seriously ill person, or someone suffering from dementia, is in, it can change very quickly.

As you enter the room or space where your Compassionate Touch session is to take place, take a few moments to assess the environment and make any minor adjustments that might facilitate a successful session. If you are working in a hospital or nursing home room with more than one occupant, you will probably want to pull the curtain between the bed of the person you have come to see and the next bed. Explain to the person in the next bed, if he or she is alert, why you are shutting the curtain, and that you will pull it back before you leave. Never ignore other people in the room or act as if they do not exist! You may need to move a small table or a chair to gain better access to the person with whom you are working. If you are in a medical facility, do not move equipment such as oxygen tanks or IV stands without asking permission of someone on the staff.

Find out how to raise and lower the sides of the bed as well as how to mechanically or manually adjust the height of the bed itself. Hospital beds are not all alike! The mechanisms may vary from bed to bed even in the same room. If you are at all in doubt, it is wise to check with a staff person to make sure it is okay to lower the guard rails on the bed. Lower the rails on the side you are working on and then raise them again before going to the other side of the bed. Put the bed height back to its original position when your session is over, unless the person you are working with is able to do it or requests a different position.

You are essentially touching a person as soon as you enter the room where she or he is. As you work with that individual, remember that everything about you is touching the person—your hands, your voice, your eyes, your facial expressions, and even your thoughts! Resolve to consciously give your undivided and focused attention to the individual you are seeing during the entire time, and to treat that person as you would want to be treated if you were in a similar situation.

If you are a primary or relief caregiver administering Compassionate Touch to a patient or to a loved one, arrange to spend a certain amount of undistracted time with that person in this particular experience of nurturing. Although you may be touching and caring for your loved one in various ways throughout the day, treat this time as special and focus your attention solely on him or her as you use specific techniques that are not necessarily a part of more general physical care and treatment.

Protecting Yourself and the People You Touch

It is essential to wash your hands thoroughly with soap and water before you begin a Compassionate Touch session, and when you are finished. It might also become necessary to wash your hands during a session. If you are seeing a number of people sequentially in the same facility, pay particular attention to this cleansing as you move from one resident to the next. Washing your hands before a session protects the individual who is susceptible to infection and washing your hands after a session protects you and the person you touch next. In most medical or extended care facilities, you will find a sink with disinfectant soap in each room, or at least in a nearby hallway bathroom. If you are moving from room to room, you can move to the next room to wash your hands there before beginning the new session. On a subtle level this may help the person you are about to work with feel that you are being careful in protecting him or her (which you are) and avoids the possibility of making the last person you worked with feel that you think his or her body is dirty or disgusting to you.

Remember that if you have not washed your hands carefully and thoroughly (working up a good lather with the soap and taking several minutes to cover every inch of both hands and forearms) and/or you have any kind of open lesion, contagious rash, cold, or infection, you are putting the person you are about to touch at risk.

Certain physical conditions would preclude massage where that condition exists. In cases of thrombosis or thrombophlebitis (inflamation of a vein) in the leg, you should avoid any pressure, with or without stroking, but you could still administer attentive touch. If you are unsure, in any situation, make certain that you have the permission of a doctor who understands your work.

You may also need to work on top of, or reach underneath, bed covers, or outer layers of clothing, to administer massage to an older person who chills easily. I used to see one ninety-eight-year old gentleman who usually wore a woolen hat, neck scarf, and sweater over his other clothing no matter what the weather, and sometimes had on several layers of clothing when he was in bed underneath his covers!

Use common sense in avoiding direct contact with lesions, undiagnosed rash or contagious skin problems. Never massage directly on an open wound,

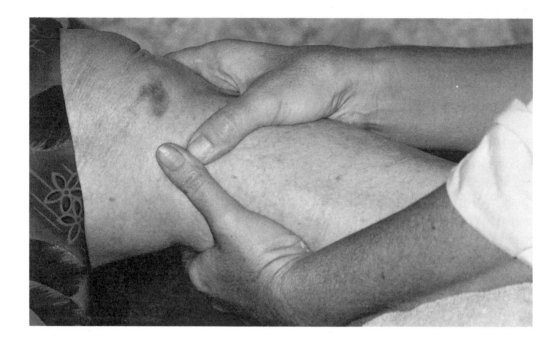

weeping rash, laceration, protrusion, or new scar tissue. Work gently around or above such conditions, holding your hands slightly above the area, focusing your attention and energy on it.

Protecting yourself energetically or psychically is also a good idea before you begin interacting with another in any kind of physical way. This may sound mystical but it is actually quite practical. Some people can quite easily "take on" another person's physical and/or emotional state of being. I learned very early on in my massage practice that if I did not consciously guard against it, I would often be experiencing whatever symptoms my client was manifesting by the end of our work together. This included physical complaints such as stomach and headaches as well as emotional states such as anxiety or depression. There are various ways to solve this problem. The grounding and centering exercises suggested in Chapter Three will help. You can visualize yourself surrounded by a golden or white light, or protected inside an invisible bubble or band of energy. Even better, you can access the source of light from within yourself and then see or feel that light growing and expanding until it radiates outward from your body. You might also repeat a short affirmation or prayer of protection. Or, you can simply make a conscious decision before you begin touching someone not to take on that person's physical symptoms, emotional feelings, or mental attitudes.

Another aspect of taking care of yourself is to insure your own comfort while working. By doing this, you will avoid unnecessary pain and fatigue, and you will be able to give your energy and full attention to the patient. If you are standing, be sure to keep your knees slightly bent rather than "locked." Bring the bed up to a workable height so that you don't have to bend over, or figure out a way to sit down while you work. Keep breathing!

During my initial visit to one chronically ill patient, I put my body in various awkward positions in order to touch this person when it was completely unnecessary to do so. I was simply too self-conscious to ask questions concerning the patient's mobility or even to ask for a chair to sit on. I stood for awhile working over the bed rails when they didn't release easily, and eventually I got on my knees and reached between the bars. I stretched my upper body over a table that could have been moved and generally made things difficult for myself in any number of ways. I was physically exhausted after I left and needed a massage to recover! I have never repeated that particular mistake!

During the Session

As mentioned before, make yourself aware of the physical limitations of the person with whom you are working. Some infirm people are able to walk slowly by themselves or with help and may prefer to see you while sitting in a favorite chair (a recliner chair works quite well if one is available) or lying on a sofa. If you are working with the frail elderly and/or the chronically ill, many people you see will be confined to a bed or a wheelchair. Some will be able to sit up or turn over and some will not. Again, adapting yourself and the techniques you use to the situation as you find it is the key!

Pain is frequently communicated through nonverbal behavior. In working with those in later life stages, you must learn to look for these nonverbal indicators of discomfort. One good way of assessing discomfort is to watch the breathing pattern of the person who you are massaging. Someone who is acutely stressed, anxious, and/or in pain will usually exhibit irregular breathing. The person may seem to hold his or her breath at intervals and/or take very long and deep breaths. The breathing may become so shallow that it is difficult to tell whether inhalation and exhalation is occurring. A person may suddenly breathe very rapidly and deeply, almost to the point of hyperventilating. As a person relaxes you will notice the breathing pattern become more normal. Someone may switch from chest to abdominal breathing. A person may yawn or let out a long sigh, after which the inhalation and exhalation of breath will become more regular and even.

As a Compassionate Touch practitioner you need to train yourself to pick up on cues as to what kind of pain is being experienced and where it may be coming from. A patient may be unable to answer the question "Does it hurt here?" or "Is this area tender?" and so you must rely on observation and intuition.

Placing a hand ever so gently directly on or just above an area of the body that is swollen, discolored, inflamed, bruised, or contracted can sometimes be enough to bring some degree of relief to the person in pain. That individual feels perceived, feels acknowledged, and experiences a moment of compassion and caring from another individual. The person then relaxes just a little, perhaps breathes a bit easier, and the discomfort is reduced, at least momentarily. That person feels that he or she does not have to bear the pain all alone. Another individual is willing to "receive" it and that actually does make a difference.

The person with whom you are working may or may not be able to communicate verbally. Some people in later life stages are simply too weak to speak or may wish to talk only with certain people. Occasionally a family member or a health care provider will tell you that someone is unable to talk or is verbally incoherent, yet during your visit that person will speak to you in perfectly understandable words. Use your best intuitive sense in deciding whether or not to tell the family member about such an occurrence. It is possible that the patient has something to communicate but simply cannot say it to a loved one, or senses that the family member is not ready to hear it. If you tell the family member your experience, that person may feel hurt that a loved one is talking to a "stranger" and yet remains silent around her or him. The caregiver may then become angry and aloof toward the patient or, more likely, toward you. Try to ascertain the effect it could have to pass this information along and whether or not it would actually be helpful to do so, before you make a decision. Encourage family members to keep communicating with their loved one, in both verbal and non-verbal ways, even if that person does not reply or seems not to hear.

I remember sitting with a woman who had been battling cancer for a long time. She had endured surgery, chemotherapy, and radiation treatments and had eventually been told by her doctors that nothing more could be done to arrest the progression of her disease. The second time I visited her in her home she was very still and quiet. We were alone in her bedroom together and at one point she seemed to summon up all her energy in order to speak. She verbalized that she just didn't see how she could do anything more. She nodded when I acknowledged that she must be very tired. I understood her to mean that she had done all she could to stay alive and that she was ready to die. It seemed as if she simply needed to get that communication across to someone. Perhaps it was easier for her to say those words to me, a relative stranger, than to her husband or to her adult children. Though her family seemed prepared to let her go, I suspect it was easier for me to tell her that she needn't do anything more, that she could rest. Without communicating anything more verbally, this lady died peacefully in her sleep a day or two later.

You may be asked to work with someone who does not speak the same language that you speak. If the person is communicative and conversant, try to have someone who does speak that person's language inform him or her that you speak only (whatever language you speak). If you find it necessary to ask the patient a question, you could use that same person as a translator. In most situations like this, things will go fine since touch is a universal language; and you will often find other ways to communicate without a common spoken language.

I work with one bedridden yet extremely expressive woman who speaks Italian and very little English. The first few times I visited this lady, I felt somewhat frustrated about this language barrier and wondered if I should learn some Italian so we could communicate. Over the months, however, we have developed a way of conversing that includes a lot of reflective feedback in the form of facial and bodily expressions and gestures, and we have no trouble communicating our fondness for each other.

In a situation where a patient obviously wants to speak and cannot but is able to write, you can try using a chalkboard or writing pad to facilitate the communication. I work with a young man who has cerebral palsy and is unable to form words in an understandable way. We talk to each other through his communications book, which contains pages of often used words and phrases as well as all the letters of the alphabet. I can ask if he is ready for his massage or if he wants his back rubbed and he can point to"Yes" or "No" in the booklet that I hold in front of him.

If you are administering Compassionate Touch to someone who is unable to speak, because of a stroke, for instance, always tell the person who you are and why you are there. Even if a person is in a comatose state, explain from time to time what you are doing. People have been known to come out of comas or to recover from strokes and to remember everything that was said and done while they were unable to respond.

I have been seeing one woman in a convalescent home twice a week for over a year. This woman, who had a stroke shortly before I began seeing her, is not able to speak and, in fact, she sometimes sleeps through our sessions. At other times, however, she reaches for my hand and looks at me directly for long periods of time. Occasionally, she makes some sounds as if trying to speak.

In this type of situation you must learn to look for subtle signs of both positive and negative responses, and signs of relaxation. I would consider a response to my presence or touch to be:

eyelids flickering or opening
eyes moving and/or head turning towards me
eyes following movement
making eye contact
change in breathing pattern
making physical contact
making any sound or moving lips as if to speak
smiling
laughing or giggling
winking
blushing
crying
stretching or moving

Positive indicators of a relaxation (or letting go) response might include:

a deep breath or sigh
a clenched fist opening
change in breathing from chest to belly
passing gas
specific muscle softening
uncrossing arms or legs
yawning
mouth opening and/or jaw dropping
falling asleep
snoring (indicating deeper sleep)

Negative indicators could include:

clenching of fists
lips or jaw tightening
crossing arms or legs
flinching
muscles tightening
facial grimacing
turning body away

Some responses that might be positive or negative, depending upon the person and the circumstances:

laughing or crying
opening or shutting eyes
gesturing
coughing
sounds

As you work with those who are nonverbal, you will learn through experience and through focusing your attention on each individual what these subtle signals mean. There will also be times when all you can do is open your heart and your hands and trust your own intuition to guide you.

In offering hands-on care to those in later life stages, you will at some point find yourself working around various kinds of medical equipment and apparatus. Feeding tubes, catheters, IV's, oxygen tubes, aspirators, monitors, and other devices may be attached to the person you are working with. In the beginning such apparatus can be distracting, even frightening. It is helpful to educate yourself as to the function of the medical equipment that the person you are massaging may be dependent upon. This is an area in which your creativity and flexibility will be helpful. You will need to adapt your massage techniques and invent new ways of working as you go along. There is almost always more than one way to accomplish a goal. It is also possible that certain devices might be unhooked for the short time you will be working with the person. It never hurts to ask.

If you are doing whole body massage, you may also need to work your way around diapers, bandages, dressings, narcotic patches, and so on. Avoid any direct pressure on narcotic patches, bandages, or dressings. If you are using long strokes on the legs and/or thighs, you may want to untape the side of a diaper in order to massage the buttocks. Do this only with the patient's permission or if requested. Proceed nonintrusively and with respect for the privacy of the individual at all times.

Loss of control over one's life, on many different levels, is usually a major issue for a rapidly aging and/or seriously ill person. One must submit to all kinds of intrusive, uncomfortable, undignified, and even embarrassing procedures in the course of diagnosis and treatment of a life-threatening illness. Nearly everyone experiences some loss of privacy and individuality during a stay in a medical facility where there are numerous rules and regulations, and where everything is done according to a strict time schedule based on keeping a large institution functioning smoothly, rather than according to individual desires or wishes. Whatever a person's professional position, status, or social standing may be outside of such institutions, everyone is treated the same inside.

Residents of any health care facility are, for the most part, largely relegated to following someone else's schedule. Their choices are greatly limited. They are often in a room with two or three other people they have never met before, and sometimes the roommates keep changing. They have little privacy. They are sometimes treated as objects or as if they do not really exist. I have observed men and women in such facilities struggling to maintain their dignity as they experience their personal power slowly slipping away. One of the most compassionate things you can do for people in such situations is to give them as much autonomy and control as possible during the time you spend with them. Let the hospital patient or nursing home resident know that he or she is "the boss." Ask permission to call people by their first name, sit on their bed, or to move personal articles. Offer simple choices as often as you can.

Avoid the temptation to do things for people that they can do for themselves. Ask people if they need help getting into bed or getting a glass of water instead of assuming that they do. Ask those with whom you are working (rather than the caregivers or family members) what they want in regard to the time you spend with them. Avoid making assumptions about and/or choices for people if they are able to communicate with you in any way.

Honor the choices of your clients, loved ones, or friends whenever possible. Let them set the tone for your special time together. If those you are working with are able to communicate well, let them lead the conversation and talk about whatever may be important. Give an opinion only if you are asked directly and refrain from lengthy "sharing" of your own experiences and points of view. Ask uncomplicated questions and then be quiet and listen!

I have sometimes given Compassionate Touch sessions over a period of time to people in their homes and then visited those same people in hospital or nursing homes (or vice versa). The environment of a medical or convalescent facility is quite different from the home environment and, naturally, certain adjustments must be made. The most obvious change in moving from a home into a medical setting, other than the unfamiliar surroundings, is the one mentioned above concerning scheduling and personal desires. This affects you as well, because you will need to check with a staff person as to when the best time for your visit might be. After you've consulted with someone in authority at the facility, always ask the resident/patient, or have the staff person ask, if you are telephoning, if that time is okay for him or her.

You may observe noticeable changes in people's behavior or attitudes when they are shifted to a new or different environment. The move itself may have been painful or otherwise traumatic. Certain things may seem easier or more difficult in one environment or the other. Family members may have varied positive or negative reactions to the change in location of their loved one. Avoid getting caught in the middle of family conflicts. Remain positive in your interactions with all the people involved. Give your opinion only if specifically requested. Remember that you can acknowledge a communication without agreeing with it. Never invalidate someone's personal experience or feelings.

In offering Compassionate Touch to those in later life stages, you may be working with people who have no relatives or close friends, or whose loved ones are too far away to visit often. In some cases, you are acting as a surrogate for those missing family members or close friends. Treat those people whom you touch as sensitively and *care*-fully as you would want someone to treat you, or someone close to you, in a similar situation.

I have learned through experience that it is best to be open to the unexpected when working with people who may be mentally confused and disoriented. It is good to remember that age, discomfort, medications, and loneliness can evoke behavior in people that is not always appropriate or rational.

Sexual Energy

It is possible that, at some point, while you are administering therapeutic massage or attentive touch, a person will become sexually aroused. This energy may manifest itself more obviously in men, but it occurs in females also. This is a natural reaction, especially when you are working with people who may have been deprived of gentle, nurturing touch for an extended period of time. You need not judge or negate the experience. On the other hand, you must be very clear about your own intentions and boundaries in your relationship with those whom you touch.

It may be necessary to verbalize restrictions regarding sexual boundaries to someone who is confused. If the person is mentally alert and able to speak, you can address the issue of sexual energy directly. You can acknowledge the deprivation that the person must be feeling and let him or her know that the feelings are okay and acceptable, and that you understand how frustrating it must be to be unable to act on those impulses. Your acknowledgement, acceptance, and understanding will go far toward alleviating that frustration and helping the person to feel satisfied by the contact you can offer.

One quite elderly gentleman whom I see regularly, who happens to be blind, occasionally exposes himself or begins to masturbate while I am giving him a back or a foot massage. When this occurs, I simply mention that he seems to need some privacy, that I will see him on my next visit, and I leave the room. I have learned, in this particular case, that the situation is less likely to arise if I time my visits early in the day when he is most awake and alert.

Respect the individuality of each person you come in contact with. Put aside images or ideas you may have about how people should behave when they are seriously ill or nearing the end of their life's journey. Put aside your mental pictures of how you would want one of your loved ones to act, or how you think you might act in a similar situation. Remain open to each individual as you encounter him or her and to each experience as it unfolds. Do your best to simply accept things the way they actually are and carry on.

HIV Disease

If you are administering therapeutic massage to seriously ill people with infectious diseases or compromised immune systems, it is important to understand the facts of how such diseases are spread. This will enable you to take appropriate precautions if necessary so that your attention can remain on the person with whom you are working rather than on your fear of becoming infected with a deadly virus.

AIDS is the worst consequence in the progression of the Human Immunodeficiency Virus known as HIV. There is, at the present time, no known cure for AIDS. The virus does not necessarily cause AIDS in everyone who is infected, and some manifestations of HIV infection remain mild for many years.

For HIV infection to occur, three things must happen simultaneously:

1. the virus must have a **proper environment** to survive
2. a sufficiently **large quantity** of the virus has to enter the system
3. there must be a **port of entry**

The HIV virus cannot pass through intact, undamaged skin. It is transmitted only when the blood, or certain body fluids, of an infected person come into direct contact with the blood or body fluids of an uninfected person. The HIV virus is found in sufficient quantities to cause infection in blood, semen, vaginal fluids, and, occasionally, in breast milk. HIV has been found in tears, sweat, and, rarely, in saliva in smaller concentrations. No case of HIV infection has been proven to have been transmitted from tears, sweat or saliva. HIV can be transmitted from one human body to another through blood to blood contact such as unclean IV needles, or open wounds in both people, and through unprotected sex.

It is good to keep a pair of vinyl or latex examination gloves (purchased in bulk at medical supply stores) handy in case they are needed. If you are likely to come into contact with blood (including bloody feces or bloody vomitus) or other bodily fluids, that may contain the HIV virus, during the course of your interaction with a client, or in the unlikely event a person should start bleeding or spitting up blood in the middle of a session, you can put on the gloves before proceeding. Remember that gloves are used as an additional, or secondary, layer of protection beyond the protection afforded by intact skin and thorough hand washing.

It is necessary to wear gloves during a massage session only if:

- you have a cut, open sore, scratches, abrasions, or a contagious rash on your hands;
- you aren't sure if your skin is intact and you might be coming into direct contact with blood or bodily fluids, or secretions that might contain blood such as urine, feces, or vomitus;
- a person has weeping herpes lesions near an area you will be touching;
- the person you are touching requests that you wear gloves;
- you do not feel comfortable touching the person without wearing gloves.

Use a sterile glove if there is concern about a patient's susceptibility to infection. Double gloving is possible if extra protection is thought to be necessary. Gloves should be disposed of after each use.

There is a product called DermaPlus that is used in professional and industrial work places to provide an antimicrobial barrier on the skin. It is a non-greasy, nontoxic barrier, which is invisible once it is rubbed on and which provides protection without affecting the sense of touch or mobility. DermaPlus comes out of a can in foam form much like shaving cream and can also be used as a secondary barrier for hands with intact skin that have been thoroughly washed.

If you have a scratch, hangnail, or infected skin area on the end of a finger, you can wear a finger cot on that particular finger. Boxes of latex finger cots can be purchased in drug stores. Each box contains several sizes so that you will be able to find one that will fit snugly wherever you need it.

In any contagious situation where direct physical contact with someone creates a health danger or does not feel comfortable to either of the two people involved in a massage session, it is possible for the practitioner to give a massage wearing surgical gloves. You can also use a number of massage techniques working with a sheet or thin blanket acting as a shield between your hands and the body you are touching. Skin on skin contact is preferable. Being touched through gloves or over covers is certainly better than being deprived of touch and many Compassionate Touch techniques and benefits remain effective.

If you are working on a continuing basis with people who are manifesting symptoms of HIV disease or AIDS, it will be important to familiarize yourself with the characteristics of the common opportunistic infections that attack such people. Such knowledge will give you a better understanding of the physical changes that occur and will guide you in taking the necessary and appropriate precautions for each one. Irene Smith describes each of these conditions in detail in her material on *Guidelines for the Massage of AIDS Patients.*

- Pneumocystis carinii pneumonia (PCP)
- Toxoplasmosis
- Cryptococcal meningitis
- Candida
- Cytomegalovirus (CMV)
- Herpes (all forms, including shingles, are highly contagious)
- Kaposi's Sarcoma (KS) — a cancer whose reddish, purple lesions may manifest externally on the body

Although every body system is different, some of the more common effects of AIDS include:

- lowered resistance to infection
- loss of appetite
- unexplained weight loss
- chronic low grade fever
- chronic fatigue and weakness
- severe diarrhea
- persistent mouth ulcers and sores
- chronic cough and other respiratory symptoms

Many people with AIDS manifest some neurological dysfunction during later stages of the disease. These can include severe headaches, blurred vision, memory loss, and personality changes. Communication skills become especially important in working with people suffering from dementia and neurological impairments; and touch becomes significant as a communication aid, in addition to its other benefits.

It is important for caregivers to understand that a diagnosis of HIV disease or AIDS often causes intense emotional reactions. In addition to the sadness and fear that most people diagnosed with any life-threatening disease experience, there may be anger at the unfair treatment of some people with AIDS and/or guilt about past actions or about the possibility of having spread the disease. There may also be a noticeable lack of support from family members or friends once the diagnosis is known.

I have worked with several AIDS patients whose families disowned or deserted them when their illness became known, out of judgement, fear and/or ignorance. One woman's companion of seven years simply disappeared one day, apparently unable to cope with her diagnosis. These kinds of things seldom happen when someone is diagnosed with inoperable cancer.

It has been my experience that people afflicted with AIDS are particularly responsive to and appreciative of therapeutic massage and touch. Along with its other benefits, massage speaks to a profound psychological need that is operative in many people suffering from HIV disease. Because of fear, igno-rance, and the lack of education in our society about how AIDS is transmitted, many people, including some health care workers, are afraid to touch, or even be in the same room with, a person who has AIDS. I could hardly believe it when a young computer analyst told me, as I massaged his hands, that during his stay in one nursing facility, he asked a health care worker for Kleenex only to have a box thrown at him from across the room! This same individual, who had beautiful, soft, smooth skin characteristic of many Afro-American people and no open lesions of any kind, commented that whenever he *was* touched, it was always with gloved hands. When the message "you are untouchable" is con-stantly being transmitted, self-esteem can begin to weaken and feelings of deprivation and isolation increase.

If you are offering massage to people with AIDS, and questions or concerns arise for you while working with them, be honest with yourself, and with those you are caring for, about your concerns. Call your local Infection Control Center or AIDS Hotline for answers to any questions that may come up. Talk with other people who work in a hands-on way with those who have HIV infection or AIDS to help alleviate your concerns and strengthen your confidence.

Ending the Session

Ideally, a Compassionate Touch session is open-ended in terms of time. It is over when both you and the person you are working with feel satisfied that the session is complete. You might spend ten minutes with the person or you might spend an hour or even longer. Much of the time, however, and for various reasons, you will probably be working within scheduled time slots, so it is important to pace yourself and to set certain guidelines.

When you begin your Compassionate Touch session, whether you are offer-ing your services on a volunteer or on a paid basis, if you have contracted for a specific length of time, remind the person you are working with how long the session will be. If the person you are seeing wants you to stay longer and if you have the flexibility to stay longer, you can offer that option and give the person a choice. If you are charging a fee for your services, you need to be clear in your own mind as to whether you are offering to extend the session on a volunteer basis or on a paid basis. If you are ambivalent about this, it will introduce unclarity and confusion into the relationship and it will affect your work together.

If you are working with someone whom you experience as being particularly "needy," you need to be very clear about your own boundaries without making the other person wrong. Some people feel so isolated and starved for companionship that they will do almost anything to keep your attention on them, and no matter how long you stay, it will never seem like long enough. Other people, frustrated by what they may experience as a loss of control over their lives, become demanding and manipulative in an effort to regain some control over something, or someone. Some people see themselves as victims and are constantly on the lookout for a savior. Such people provide us with opportunities to examine our motivations for doing what we do, to grow in our ability to communicate clearly, to remain centered in who we are, and to be open to others without judging them.

I once heard a story about an experiment carried out in a large medical institution. A doctor went from room to room visiting with patients. Shortly after the doctor left the room, each patient was asked "How long did the doctor spend with you?" The patients all said that the doctor had spent at least fifteen minutes, maybe more, with them. In fact, this doctor had spent exactly five minutes with each person. It was concluded that the patients felt the doctor had spent much longer with them than he actually had because he a) pulled up a chair and sat down beside them; b) looked them in the eyes; and, c) held their hands. In other words, this man positioned himself so that he and the patient were at the same eye level, focused his attention on them, and reinforced his attention with physical contact! If you develop the ability to be consciously present, giving people your full and undivided attention while you are with them, then those people will feel satisfied at the end of your visit. Whatever length of time you spend with them, those people will seldom be left wishing you could have stayed longer.

When the time you have allotted for a session is nearing an end, tell the person you are with that you have a few more minutes to stay and, if possible, find out what that person would like from you in those few minutes. This gives the person you are working with an opportunity to ask for something specific or to say whatever may be on his or her mind before you must leave.

Remember to restore the environment to the way it was when you came into the session. If you feel there is a very good reason for changing something, ask the resident of the room before doing so. Put stockings, and/or slippers that you may have removed back on. If you have taken off someone's watch, remember to replace it. Be sure that you put the watch back on the same arm and in the same position in which you found it. I once noticed that I had put a gentlemen's watch back on his arm in the reverse direction so that the face of his watch was upside down and not easily readable. This may seem like a little thing, but it can be quite frustrating to someone who has been partially paralyzed by a stroke or who has barely enough strength to lift an arm. It is particularly important to put bed trays back in the same position so that familiar and needed items may be easily reached.

As previously mentioned, remember to return the side rails of hospital beds to their up position if that is the way they were when you arrived. If someone in a health care facility asks you to leave the bed rails in the down position, tell that person you must check with someone in charge before doing so. If you were to leave the guard rails down and the patient subsequently fell out of bed and was hurt, not only would you have to deal with your own feelings of responsibility in the matter, but both you and the facility could be found negligent in a lawsuit!

If you have been working with someone in a wheelchair, ask where he or she would like to be positioned before you leave. You might need to push that person back to a recreation area, for instance, or to a dining hall. If the person you have been working with is communicative, tell that person that you are locking the wheels on her or his chair in place, unless you know the person is able to move the chair without help.

When working with residents of convalescent or extended care facilities, never remove the safety belt on a wheelchair or try to help someone move from a chair into a bed or vice versa! If a person makes such a request, explain that you are not on the staff of the facility and you are not authorized to do such things, but that you will relay the request to someone who does work there, and be sure you do relay the information.

You may notice sudden changes in the mood, demeanor, or desires of the people you work with. It is important to remember that the aging process can include many physical changes that require emotional adjustment. Age-related changes, which often occur gradually, may include a decline in mental acuity, agility, mobility, and stamina. Changes in vision and hearing and mild memory loss are common in the aging process. Medications can also contribute to disorientation and mental confusion. I see one very dear lady, afflicted with Alzheimer's Disease, who often talks nonstop during the time I spend with her. Most of what she says is not logical or relevant to present time and space, though it seems important and meaningful to her. To me, it would seem useless and cruel to try and "correct" or re-orient this lady so I simply listen to and acknowledge whatever she has to say. This, along with being touched, seems to give her comfort and pleasure, and she always thanks me at the end of our sessions.

Do your best to simply go along with whatever is important to the person you are touching in the moments when you are with him or her, as much as you can, no matter how illogical or irrational the comments or desires may seem to you. Do what you can to accommodate any requests that are made. Realize that people will ask things of you that are beyond your jurisdiction or impossible to do. Be as clear and direct as you can in communicating what you cannot do and why. If you are unable to fulfill a request, be honest about it and try to find someone who can, or suggest an alternative. If you tell someone that you will

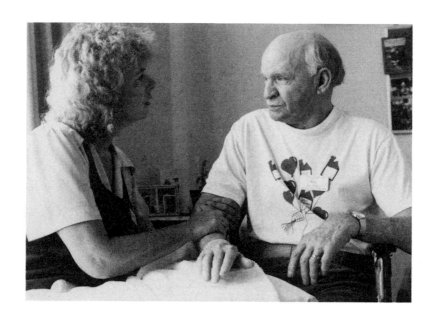

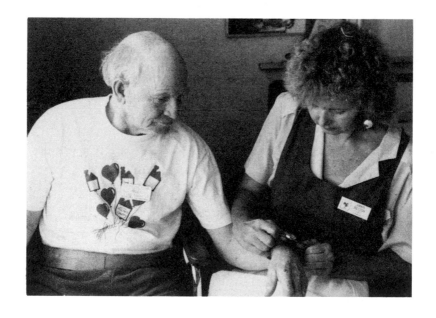

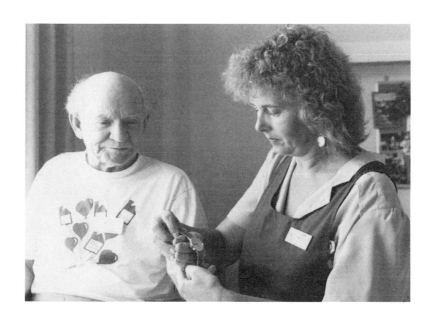

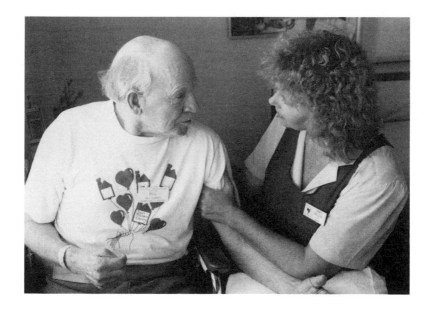

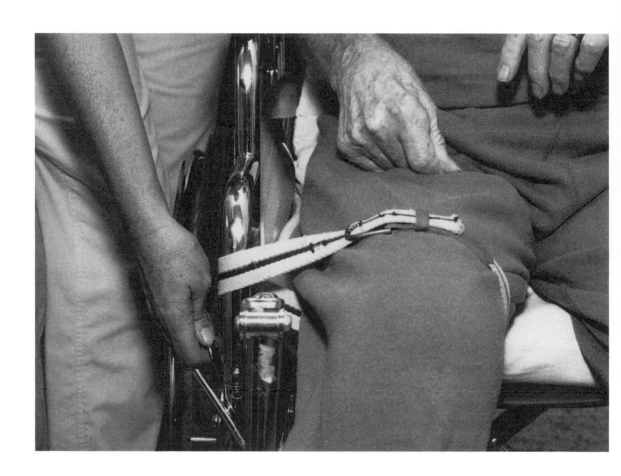

pass his or her request on to someone else such as a nurse, administrator, or family member, be sure that you follow through so that, whatever the outcome, you have kept your part of the agreement made with that person.

When Death Seems Near

When working with someone who is nearing the end of life, each time you say good-bye there is the chance that you will not see that person again. This is, of course, true for all of us at any time (and a good reason for keeping our relationships "current") yet is perhaps a bit more predictable in relationships with the seriously ill and/or those quite advanced in age. Do not leave unsaid or undone anything you feel is important in your relationship with a person when you leave after a Compassionate Touch session. You may be able to observe and sense when the end is very near and you may not. Death, like birth, seems to pick its own time to come and can sometimes occur when we least expect it to.

I worked with a particular individual over a period of seven months, weekly in the beginning and eventually twice a week. I learned to cherish this person and always looked forward to our time together. After I'd been visiting this gentleman for a month or so, I spontaneously kissed him on the cheek before I left one day and it then became an important ritual of our parting each time we were together. As my friendship with this man, and my affection for him, grew over the months, I had the impulse several times to say "I love you" to him, but for some reason I just never verbalized the thought.

As I was getting into my car to drive to this man's home one day, I had another impulse. I noticed a particular rose blooming in the garden and had the thought that I'd like to take him that rose. I then reasoned that if I took the time to go back into the house to get the clippers, and something to put the rose in to keep it fresh for the 30-minute drive, I might be late for our appointment, so I decided I would wait and take one of the roses two days later when I would be seeing him again.

I arrived at his home that day to find this patient in a slightly weaker condition and less talkative than usual. There had, however, been many ups and downs in the course of his disease and so I really didn't think too much of it. Looking back on it, I remember being reluctant to leave him at the end of our session but, as I kissed him goodbye that Tuesday morning, I said I'd see him on Thursday. After his death the next day, I regretted not having taken him the rose. And even though I know he knew it, I regretted never having told this unique individual that I loved him.

It is best to avoid the "I'll see you next week" type of goodbye when leaving someone who is nearing the end of life. It is better to say something like "I'm glad to have seen you today" or "It's been good to spend time with you."

Often, people approaching death will give you some kind of clue to indicate that they feel the time is near, or as a way of telling you goodbye. It may be something very simple or subtle, something which could be easily overlooked in a different situation.

One woman whom I worked with over a period of several weeks was in a great deal of pain and spoke very little during our last session together. She was resting in a hospital bed that had been placed in the living room of her home. I remember that she was experiencing severe headaches as well as confusion and anxiety. When it was time for me to leave, she seemed reluctant to let go of my hand and held it tightly for some minutes. Knowing her fear of being alone, I assured her that she had many people who cared about her (neighbors, church friends, and relatives had arranged a schedule so that someone was always there) and that whatever happened as things progressed, she was not going to be alone. I also assured her that we were all committed to helping her be as comfortable as possible.

As I opened the front door to leave, I turned back to look at this sweet and fragile lady who had essentially remained curled up under her blankets and facing the wall since my arrival. She turned and raised herself slightly from the bed, looked directly at me for the first time that day, and said in a relatively strong and clear voice, "Goodbye, Dawn. Have a good evening with your family." I told her I would be thinking about her. I'm sure she sensed, as I did, that we would not meet again. I was not surprised to receive a phone call less than two days later telling me she had died.

Some people who work on a continuing basis with individuals who are confronting death report that being with such people becomes almost addictive. I think one reason this occurs is because being in the presence of people who are approaching the death experience galvanizes our attention in a way that everyday life may not. It awakens us to what is actually important and real; and it keeps us focused in present time.

Another reason why spending time with such individuals may appeal to us is that we have a deep desire to unravel the Great Mystery of Life that we call Death. We have so much to learn about how to approach death and so many questions about how to die. Sitting in quiet contact with a person nearing the completion of a lifetime, sharing the fears and anticipations of someone who is about to withdraw from a dysfunctional body, witnessing the transitional moment when an individual moves from one realm of existence into another may bring us a little closer to participating in and resolving that mystery, and to experiencing life as it actually occurs. In this way, working with the dying can be challenging, exhilarating, and even liberating.

❧ 7 ❧

CAREGIVING FOR THE CAREGIVER

As a mother at risk of her life watches over her only child, so let everyone cultivate a boundlessly compassionate mind toward all beings.

The Buddha

Support for At-Home Caregivers

If you are seeing a chronically or acutely ill person in his or her home, be cognizant of the stress level of the family member, companion, or close friend who is acting as primary caregiver. This is a different situation from a trained health care professional, who is not emotionally attached to a patient, taking care of someone. Whether a person has consciously chosen to take on the responsibility of caring for a loved one at home or has simply fallen into the situation for financial or other reasons, the caregiver takes on an enormously difficult and fatiguing task. Being physically responsible for another adult is hard and demanding work. It is emotionally draining to watch someone you love decline in health and strength, knowing you can do nothing to stop the progression of a debilitating disease. Caregivers are forced to confront the pain, anger, and sadness of a loved one while coping with similar feelings within themselves. The whole process can seem like an exhausting uphill struggle.

There may be other loved ones acting as secondary or relief caregivers who are also under stress, and the relationships between these family members and caregivers may be strained. You may find yourself in the middle of a highly stressed family trying to cope with both their own and others' reactions to a situation that everyone wishes didn't exist. Family members may be in different stages of acceptance of their loved one's condition and each one may have different coping mechanisms. Try not to get caught in the middle of family discussions or disagreements or to get seduced into "taking sides." It is essential, both from a professional and a personal point of view, to remain impartial in such situations, and to give one's honest opinion, in a non-evaluative way, only if asked. Practice family therapy techniques only if you are qualified to do so and your skills in that area are specifically requested.

You may find caregivers on an emotional roller coaster, experiencing a variety of feelings including fear, anger, frustration, abandonment, grief, and loneliness, as well as love and compassion. People you encounter who are in the situation of taking care of an aging relative or a seriously ill loved one may be distressed, confused, irritable, depressed, overwhelmed, exhausted.

Caregivers often complain of physical pain in the neck and shoulder area and/or back pain. This may be due to the strain of too much or improper lifting of an increasingly immobile person. The pain may also be a way of telling others that the burden is becoming too great, the load is too heavy to carry, and that some relief is needed. In other words, the caregiver's discomfort, whether caused by physical misuse of the body or by mental and/or emotional anxiety and stress, is a warning signal and a cry for help.

You can support caregivers in various ways, in addition to offering them a back and neck rub or some other kind of therapeutic massage. A simple acknowledgement of the reality of a situation can be enormously validating for a caregiver and may be deeply appreciated. If you mentally put yourself in a caregiver's shoes for a moment, it is easy to appreciate the labor and the courage of such a person, and to honestly comment on it. Avoid saying that you understand or know how the person feels unless you yourself have actually been in the exact same situation.

If the caregiver is open to it, a gentle squeeze of the hand, an arm around the shoulder, or a touch on the heart can let the person know that you see the difficulty of the situation, that you sense his or her fatigue and level of stress. You might ask caregivers what they do to nurture themselves. You can then encourage such people to take some time while you are working with their loved one to take a walk or a shower, to do something refreshing or different, just for themselves.

Caregivers of the seriously ill often spend a good deal of their time trying to "hold things together," sometimes denying their own needs and feelings in order to be there for others. Such people may be afraid to relax even a little bit fearing that if they do, they will fall apart completely and not be able to carry on. They may sense that letting themselves be nurtured and cared for will make them feel vulnerable or bring up feelings that they are reluctant to face or accept. It is important to acknowledge and accept such fears or reluctance and not to challenge someone to move beyond what they feel they are capable of in any given moment. At the same time, one can offer support by encouraging a caregiver not to let their own needs go unmet for too long or to push themselves too hard without relief. Caregivers may be most in need, and more willing to accept Compassionate Touch in the weeks and months following the death of the loved one they are caring for.

One of the best gifts you can offer to an emotionally drained and weary caregiver is to simply listen and understand how it is for that person without imposing your own experience or opinions. Giving an individual your conscious and focused attention for just five minutes, listening with your heart as well as with your ears, can have a greater impact than you might imagine.

On-Site Massage Therapy

Health care professionals need to be encouraged to relax also. I visit one facility where a creative Director of Services helps me turn a small examining room equipped with a padded table into a massage therapy center for personnel once a month. This supervisor sometimes gives the gift of a short massage session to an employee who seems to be particularly stressed or to one who has performed especially well on the job.

An owner/administrator of several convalescent facilities once called and asked me to come to two of her nursing homes once a month as part of an employee incentive program. Her idea was that any employee who had not missed a day of work that month, or one who had come up with a useful safety idea, would have his or her name put into a bowl for a drawing to receive a fifteen minute chair massage "on the house."

I have noticed that health care seems to be a high-stress-level profession and that those who look after the health of others are sometimes in poor health themselves. I am happy to say that an increasing number of health care professionals are learning to appreciate the relaxation and stress reduction benefits of massage and touch therapy, both for their general health and for better performance on the job, and are availing themselves of stress reduction programs that include techniques such as therapeutic massage. Though therapeutic massage may be a new experience, once people experience the benefits of massage, they tend to want sessions as often as possible. Some of the health care workers to whom I give therapeutic massage sessions were once quite dubious about receiving a massage, even as a gift. Now some of them want to learn massage techniques so they can trade sessions with each other during lunch breaks!

On-site chair massages can be given right at someone's desk, as in the photographs on the following pages, or in a special room or office set aside for that purpose during your visit to a facility. A low-backed chair without arms is best because you have more access to the back of the person on whom you are working. As always, you must be ready to adapt to the situation and utilize whatever is readily available.

You can purchase special desktop-massage devices that fit over the edge of almost any desk or table. These systems include a padded surface for the chest to rest against and a padded face cradle, both of which are adjustable for height and angle. There are also massage chairs cn the market that are fairly light weight and collapse easily for moving from site to site. These padded chairs are constructed in a such a way that they allow a person to sit comfortably with the knees supported, and in a face forward, leaning position. The practitioner then has easy access to the entire back of the person sitting in the chair, as well as the head, neck, and shoulder area. If you are doing a lot of on-site chair massage work, you might want to consider one of these options. Such devices might be used in working with older or ill people who are alert and mobile as well as with staff members in health care environments.

Another option for administering on-site massage therapy to health care staff would be to create a massage table by placing a foam pad, covered with a sheet, on top of a cafeteria type table if one is available. You could also bring a portable massage table to the site and set it up in a spare room. You can then work with people lying either face down or face up on the table, using a variety of massage strokes either over clothing or directly on the skin.

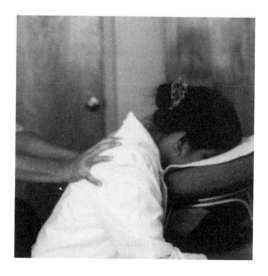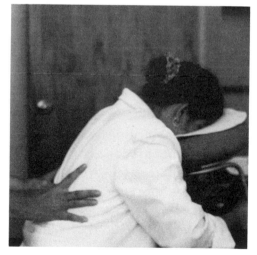

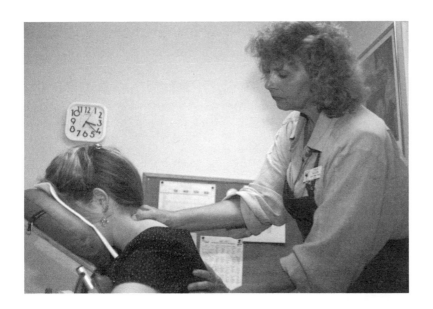

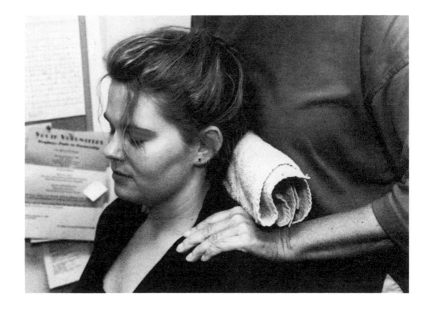

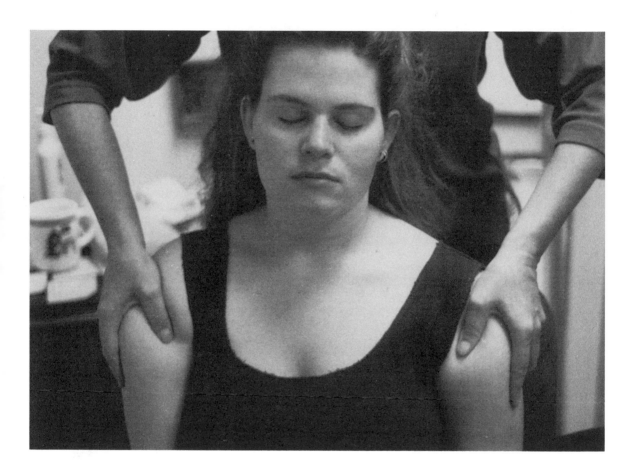

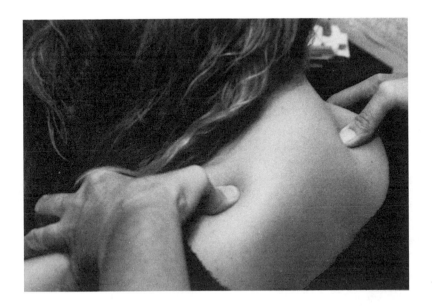

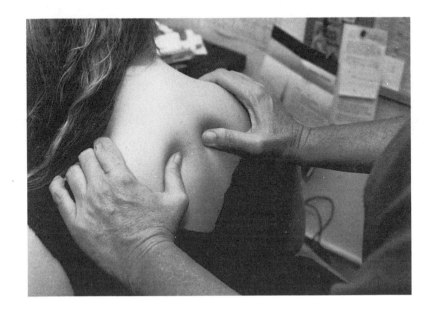

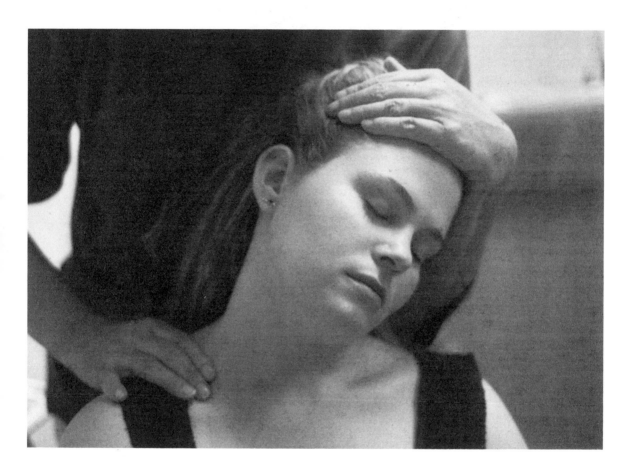

In my experience, extra space is scarce in most extended care facilities. Supervisors and even top administrators may spend their work days in converted closets and shower stalls. I have given a number of chair massages in just such windowless and cramped cubicles, with lights that couldn't be dimmed and phones that kept ringing, yet somehow recipients were able to relax during their therapeutic massage sessions, and to resume their duties feeling rejuvenated and cared for.

Self-Care

Remember to include yourself in reflecting on caring for the caregiver! This means setting limits, taking time to relax, and keeping yourself in balance physically, emotionally, and mentally. It means treating yourself with as much mercy, loving-kindness, forgiveness, and compassion as you give to those you care for.

You cannot be all things to all people all the time. There are an endless number of people in the world who would no doubt benefit from being touched attentively and compassionately. Even if you decide to administer to such people as a full-time job or spend all your spare time as a volunteer in hospitals or in care facilities for the ill and the elderly, you will be able to touch a relatively small number of those individuals. If you ignore your own needs, you will be able to work less and less productively with fewer and fewer people.

Working with people who are in crisis, who are in a great deal of pain, or who are experiencing a high level of stress and anxiety is challenging. It requires concentration. It requires focusing our attention and opening our hearts. It requires pushing through our barriers and limitations, going beyond what we think we are capable of, in order to remain present with a fellow human being who is being pushed way beyond what he or she ever thought possible or acceptable. It requires meeting our own pain with mercy as well as greeting the pain and suffering of others with mercy. If we are to be effective in serving others, we must allow our self-compassion to surface.

"Take as good care of yourself as you do of patients," exhorts one nurse/ thanatologist. In other words, give the same kind of conscious attention to your own well being as you do to those whom you serve through Compassionate Touch. Learn to comfort yourself, nurture yourself, cherish yourself, and forgive yourself. Watch for clues that will alert you to an imbalance in your life.

Unresolved stress may manifest itself in angry feelings, headaches, stomach pain, inability to concentrate, and fatigue. Typical symptoms of long-term stress can include insomnia, loss of interest in pleasurable activities, lack of sexual and/or creative energy, increasing dependence on alcohol or mood-altering drugs, depression, and increased susceptibility to common illnesses such as colds and flu.

If you are becoming irritable with or critical of your close friends and family members, if you are catching every "bug" that comes around, if you are always tired, if you are over indulging in unhealthy substances, eating constantly or forgetting to eat, unable to sleep or sleeping more than usual, it is time to stop, step back, and pay attention to what is really going on. You may want to lighten your load a bit or make a conscious effort to spend some extra time relaxing by yourself. You may need to take some time off to play with your family and friends. You cannot continue to give to others unless your own heart is nourished and your own energy is renewed and regenerated.

If you are spending a great deal of time nurturing others through physical contact and touch, make sure you are receiving nurturing touch as well. Trade sessions with another massage therapist or set up regular appointments for some type of bodywork. Do not wait until you are on overload and/or in physical pain to put your attention on your own body.

Take the time to contemplate and decide what is needed for you to maintain a balance and then, as an ongoing project, work toward creating health and harmony in your life. Try to eat well, get regular exercise, develop a philosophy of living that sustains you, and find a productive way of processing your feelings as they arise—through a support group, an art or dance class, individual or group therapy, spiritual practices, meditation, writing, music, mountain climbing, or whatever method or medium works for you. I know of one hospice caregiver who takes herself to the beach at regular intervals. She says she gives her tears to the ocean and feels calmed and replenished in return.

"Burn out" is a term used frequently these days, in professional circles, to refer to a state of total exhaustion or overwhelm. It means that one's energy is burned up, gone. Evelyn Baulch calls burn out "a bankruptcy of your physical, emotional and spiritual bank account." In a chapter devoted to the subject of burnout in her book, *Extended Health Care At Home*, she suggests that there must be as many deposits as withdrawals in one's personal account in order to maintain balance.

Dr. Dale Larson, Chairman of the Department of Counseling Psychology at Santa Clara University, echoes this sentiment in his video series on "The Caring Helper" when he points out that stress occurs when demands exceed resources. Some of the antidotes he suggests for avoiding burnout and combating stress are: setting limits; exercise; relaxation and meditation; compartmentalization; working toward specific goals; and building a support system.

If you begin to feel that you never have any time to yourself, make the decision to spend just ten or fifteen minutes per day doing something to improve your physical/mental/emotional health. It could be something as simple as a hot bubble bath every night or a walk every morning. Below is a simple relaxation exercise, which you might try for ten minutes a day.

1. Find a quiet, peaceful place away from phones and other distractions.
2. Make yourself comfortable in a sitting position.
3. Close your eyes.
4. Inhale slowly and deeply through your nose and exhale slowly blowing the air out through your mouth.
5. Let your body relax (you may want to tighten or tense and then relax different parts of your body one by one).
6. Put your attention on your breathing as you continue to inhale and exhale normally (or focus your attention in another way by silently repeating a word such as "one," or "peace" on each exhale).
7. If your attention wanders, simply bring it back to your breath or to the word you have chosen to repeat.

You can gradually increase the time you spend doing this exercise, or try doing it twice a day if you find it relaxing. I have done this exercise in my car before going in to visit a client, on airplanes, and even in a public restroom. It is often just the "pick me up" I need when I'm feeling tired or simply need to re-center myself after a particularly difficult visit with someone.

Processing Grief and Integrating Loss

Choosing to work with those who are in later life stages means that you will be confronted with dying and with death on a regular basis. Dealing with some of your own feelings and issues about aging, illness, death, and dying is an important prerequisite to practicing hands-on caregiving with the elderly and/ or the ill. It is also another way of taking care of yourself so that you can continue to care for others.

If you work a great deal with the aged and with those who are seriously ill, the reality of your experience will afford you a natural avenue to continue your own inner process in regard to your concerns and fears. Being confronted with that which is unfamiliar, uncomfortable, threatening, and even frightening offers you a tremendous opportunity for personal and spiritual growth.

Any time you open your heart to another and let that individual have personal meaning to you, you are also opening yourself to the pain of loss. A unique intimacy can develop fairly quickly between two people in the context of Compassionate Touch sessions. When a person you have been working with, even for a short period of time, dies, you will experience a loss, possibly on several levels. In addition to your sadness about the end of a particular form of relating and the knowledge that you will not see that person again, you may feel suddenly "cut off," superfluous, or unneeded. The periods of time you spent with that individual each day or week are suddenly empty. The flow of your caring energy toward that person is disrupted. You must go through a letting go process in relation to the person who has died and possibly to other people involved with that person and find new ways to channel your energy.

You may or may not be invited to attend a memorial service or asked to share in the grieving process with the family and close friends of the deceased. If you are working simultaneously with a number of people in later life stages, you will probably not have the time to attend the funeral service of each one who dies. If you are part of a volunteer organization or caregiving team, you may have the support of group meetings in which you can share your feelings with others who have experienced similar kinds of losses. If such opportunities are not available to you, find a supportive friend or loved one who is good at listening so that you can process your feelings.

If there is something you want to say to the person who has died, you can send those thoughts out mentally. You can sit down and write a letter to that person or compose a dialogue until you feel the conversation you want to have is finished. Though such exercises may seem a bit strange at first, I have found in my own grief work that these and similar techniques can be very helpful.

One "completion" exercise I have found useful, both for myself and in training others, is drawn from a Gestalt Therapy technique in which you sit down opposite another human being who, for the sake of the exercise, will represent someone you want to say something to who cannot be physically present with you. You look at the person who has agreed to do this exercise with you as if they were the person you want to talk to and you say everything you wish to say to that individual. Stay with it until you feel "complete" with that person. It may be helpful in getting started to follow a list of beginnings such as:

> *I feel angry that ...*
> *I feel sad because ...*
> *I want to tell you that ...*
> *I am glad that ...*
> *I am sorry that ...*
> *I wish ...*
> *I forgive you for ...*
> *I want to tell you ...*

Using "I" statements will help you talk about yourself and what is true for you, rather than making statements about the other person. If you cannot find someone to sit in the chair, you can put a photograph of the person you want to talk to in the chair or simply visualize the person sitting in the chair opposite you. You may need to do the exercise once a day or once a week with the same person in mind, until you feel you have really said everything you want to say to that particular individual.

This kind of exercise supports you in saying goodbye to someone you cared about who has died, to someone who has moved out of your life, or to someone with whom you find it difficult to communicate in person. Such an exercise is helpful in integrating change or loss of any kind so that you are freed to move on.

Sometimes, writing a poem or composing a song that expresses something about a person who has died, about your interaction with that individual, or about your own feelings can be helpful in the grief process. You might choose an art form such as painting, drawing, sculpting, or creating a collage to help you access, visualize, and express your emotions. These expressions can be kept private or you might decide to share them with family or friends of the deceased, or with other members of the helping community.

We must each forge our own way through trauma, change, and grief. There is no right or wrong way. The process will take as long as it takes. Our reactions will be slightly different with each loss. The death of a particular patient, friend, or client may bring back to you a loss from earlier in your life that you have not yet completely processed. You then have an opportunity for deeper healing and integration. If you are giving Compassionate Touch sessions to someone who reminds you of one of your parents or another loved one who has died, or to an individual who is suffering from the same disease as someone you have known and loved, you will probably be more emotionally reactive to that person's illness and eventual death.

When you have been relating to someone through hands-on, compassionate care and that person dies, you will feel the loss more or less intensely depending on how attached you have become to that individual. You may process your feelings fairly quickly or it may take some time. What is crucial to your continued mental and emotional health is that you acknowledge, experience, and express your reactions to the loss of that physical relationship. Ask for help if necessary and take whatever time you need. Use whatever tools you have at your disposal, to assist you in the grieving process. Denial of the emotions connected with grief can lead to disease and to any number of other physical, mental, and emotional problems.

Not long ago I was working with two different women who were suffering from the same type of cancer. Both these women were close to my own age and both had teenage children. The two women were quite different in personality and temperament, and I liked them both. I had been seeing each of these women for only a few weeks when one of them died. The next day, I made a previously unscheduled visit to see the other woman and her husband because I sensed that she, too, might die soon. As I was driving home that day, I took several wrong turns, ended up on a dead-end street, and nearly ran head-on into a large truck! When I got home I switched on the television and began eating nonstop. Later that evening, I was extremely irritable with my husband and daughter. I developed a raging headache, and I could not figure out why I was so tired!

I finally realized that I was doing everything I could to avoid experiencing the anger and the grief I was feeling—at the unfairness of this disabling disease taking women in the prime of life away from their families! My heart ached for the daughter of the woman who had died the day before, for her scientist husband, her grieving parents, and her younger sister, all of whom had been helpless against the illness that so quickly overwhelmed their gentle loved one. I felt the pain of the woman about to die, confronting her death so directly, the woman I had touched, and laughed, and cried with earlier that day. This woman was six years younger than me and I had a child in preschool! Those facts scared me. I felt threatened somehow, and vulnerable. As soon as I allowed all my feelings to surface, allowed myself to release my anger and my tears, and opened my heart to my fear and my vulnerability, my headache and fatigue disappeared!

To the extent that you are able to accept your grief and bring it into conscious thought and expression, it will dissolve. Whatever you have learned from your experience, whatever you have gained from your interaction with a particular individual, can then be integrated into your life. Your relationship with that person will contribute to and enrich your work with others.

You will find it difficult to be with another's discomfort, whether it be physical pain or mental agony, if you have not allowed yourself to open to the possibility of that same situation occurring in your own life. If you are able to face and accept your own fears and anxieties about aging, illness, death, and dying, you will be able to support someone else in facing and accepting his or her fears as they arise.

❦ 8 ❦

Compassionate Touch
In Action

The gift of life ... is no less beautiful when it is accompanied by illness or weakness ... mental or physical handicaps, loneliness or old age. Indeed, at these times, human life gains extra splendor as it requires our special care, concern and reverence.

Cardinal Terence Cooke

The photographs in this section of the book are presented without commentary or explanation, other than the first name of the person featured in each section. These photos are included here to give the reader an idea of how specific Compassionate Touch techniques, discussed earlier in the book, might be implemented in various settings with different individuals. The photos were taken during actual Compassionate Touch sessions, rather than "staged" in any way. The recipients of Compassionate Touch seen in these particular photographs range in age from forty-two to ninety-eight.

The temple bell stops
But the sound keeps coming
Out of the flowers

Basho

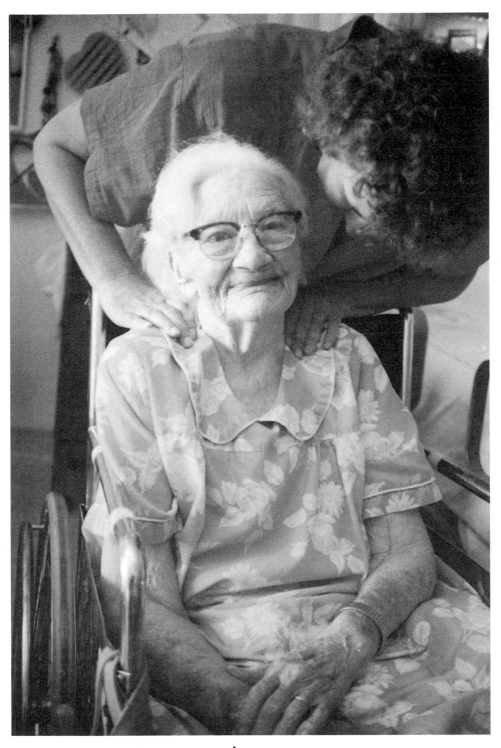

Anna

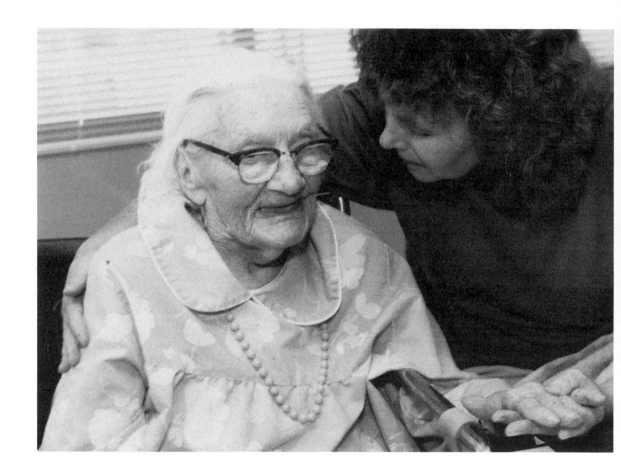

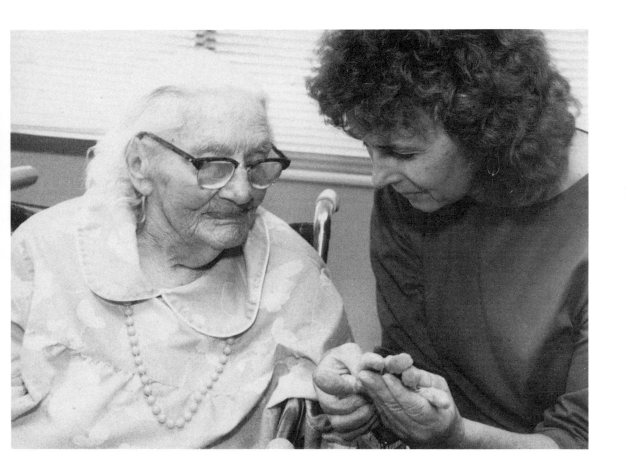

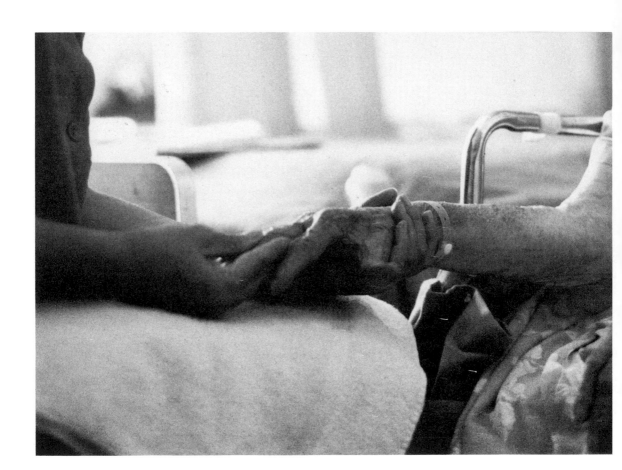

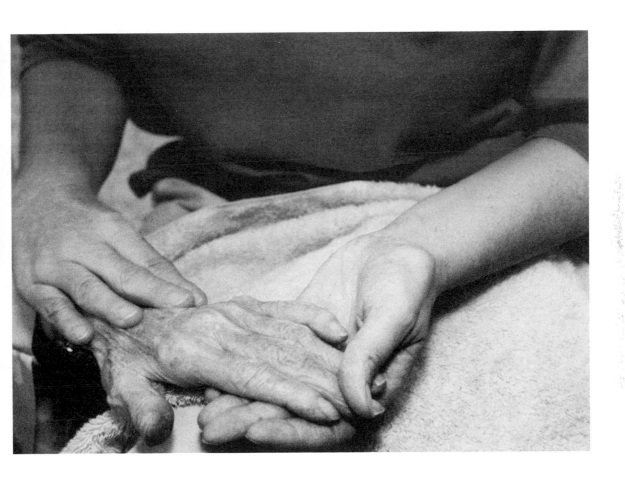

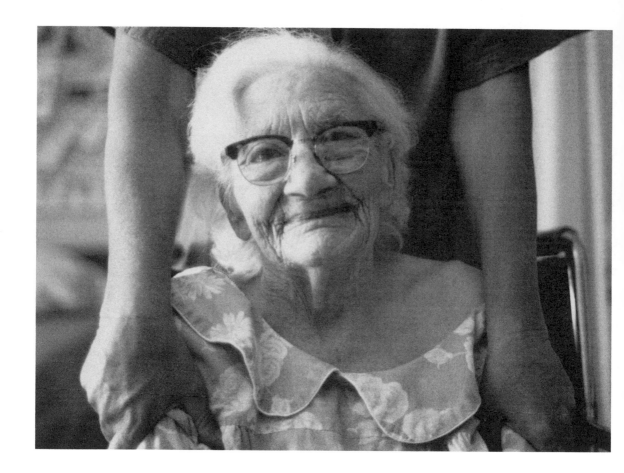

Robert

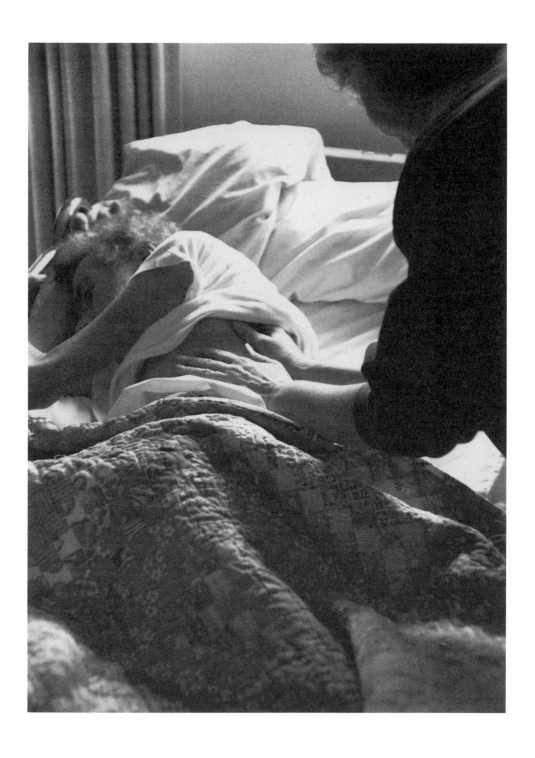

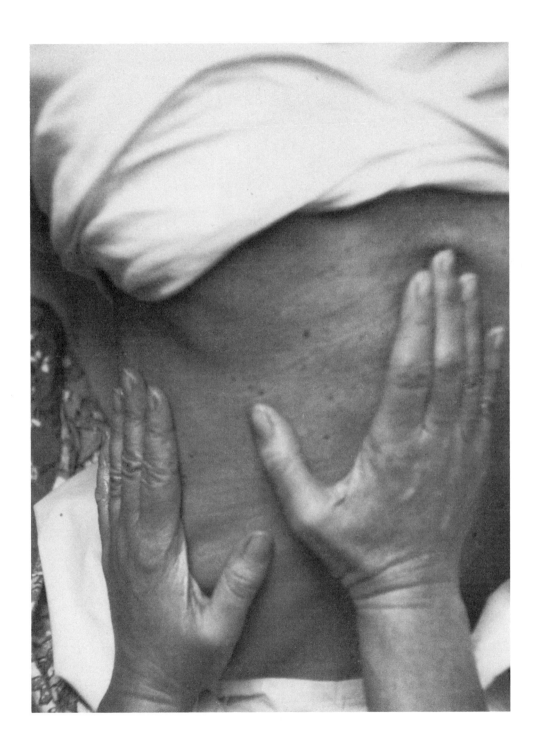

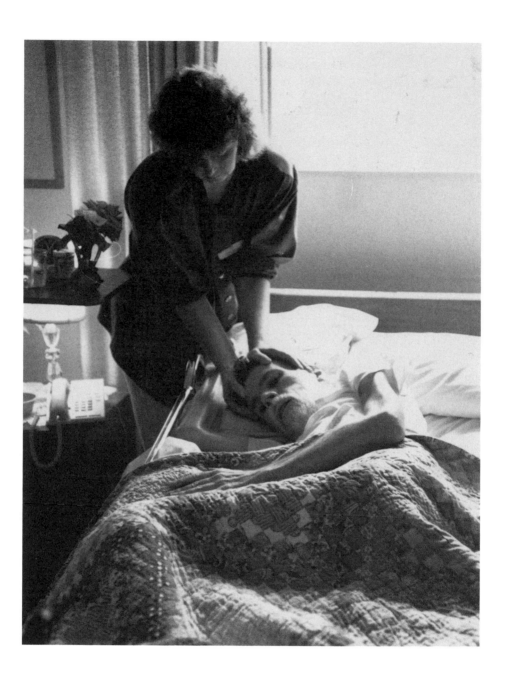

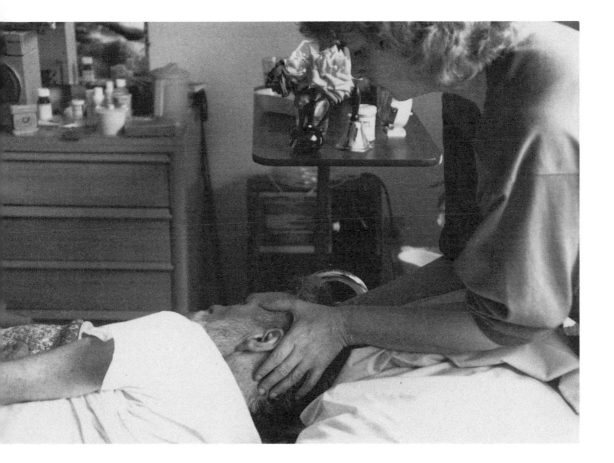

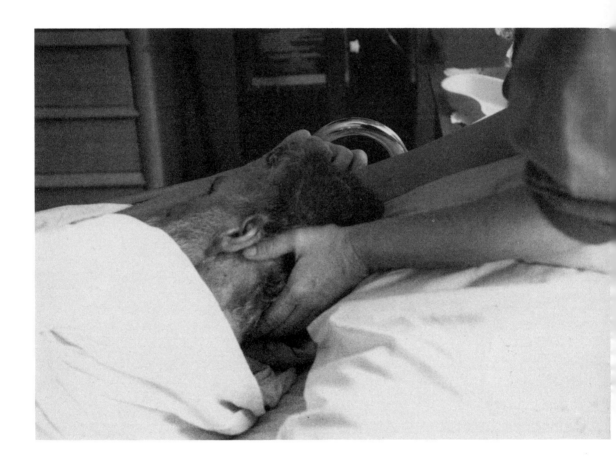

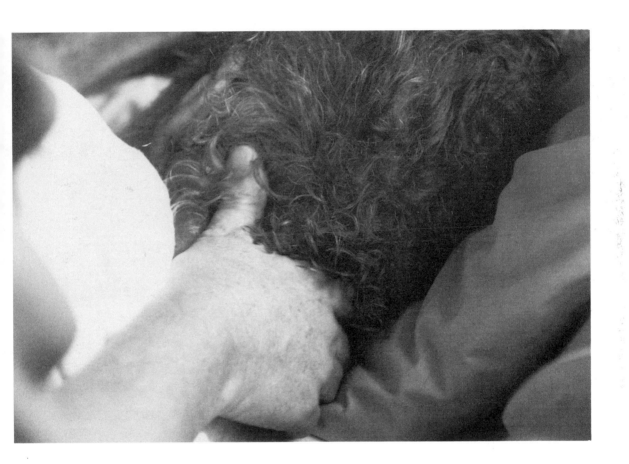

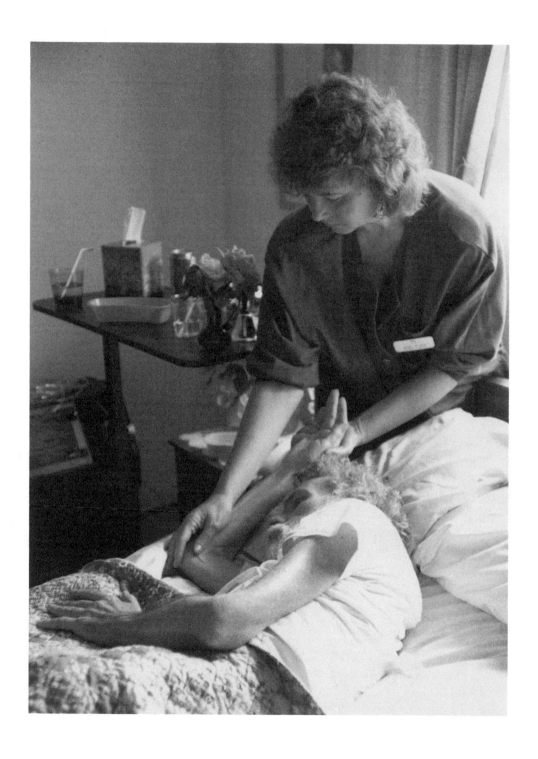

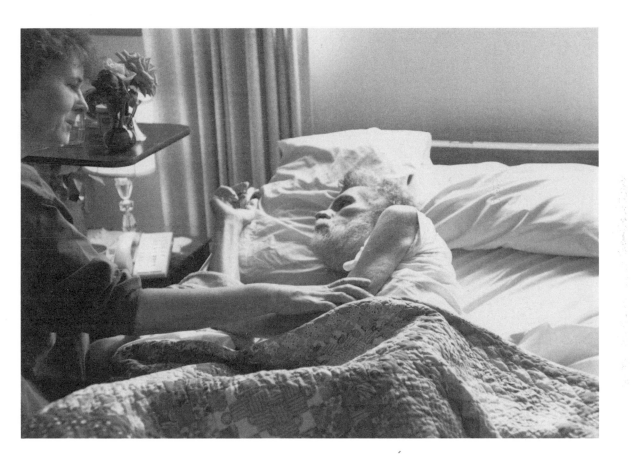

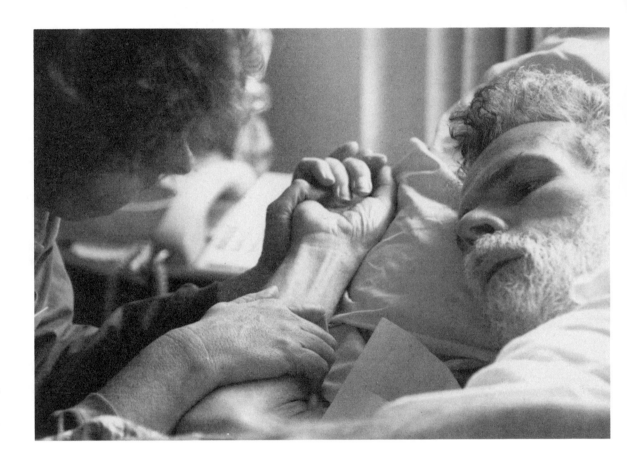

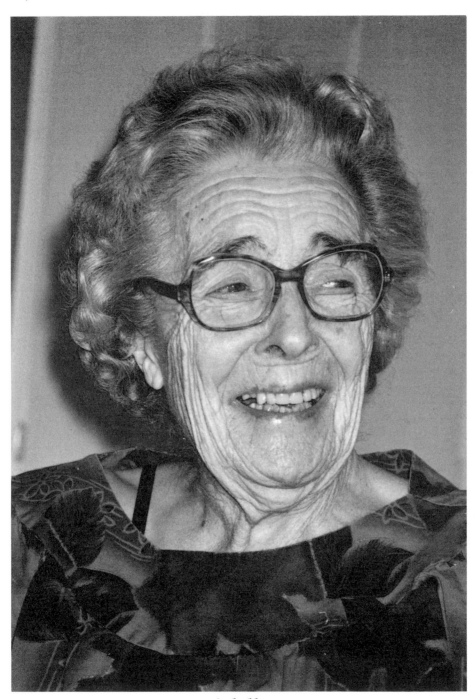

Adelle

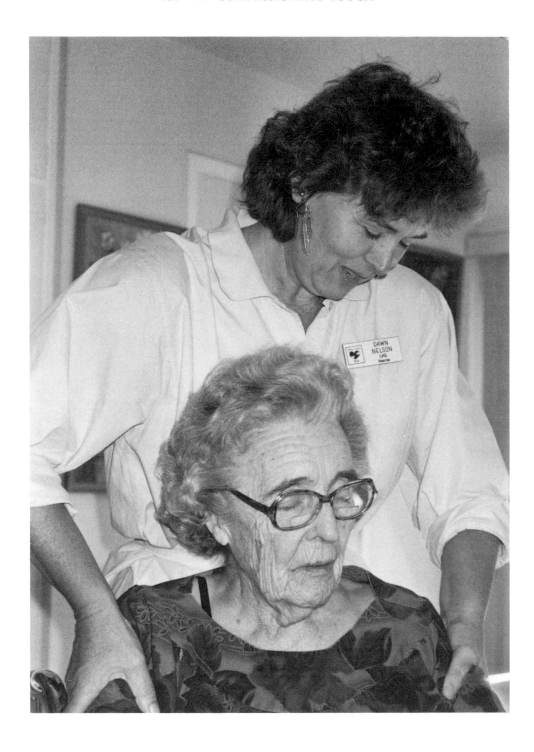

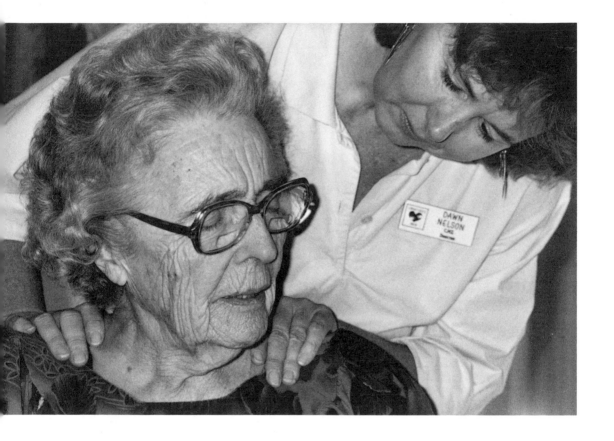

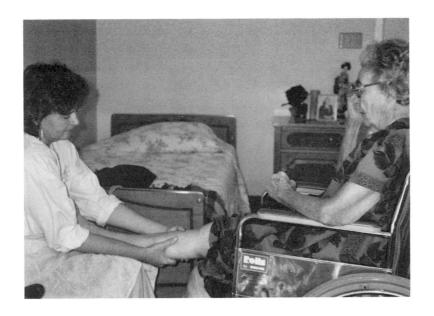

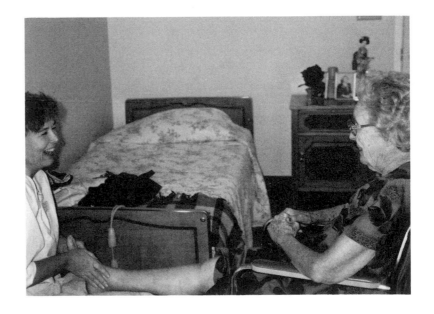

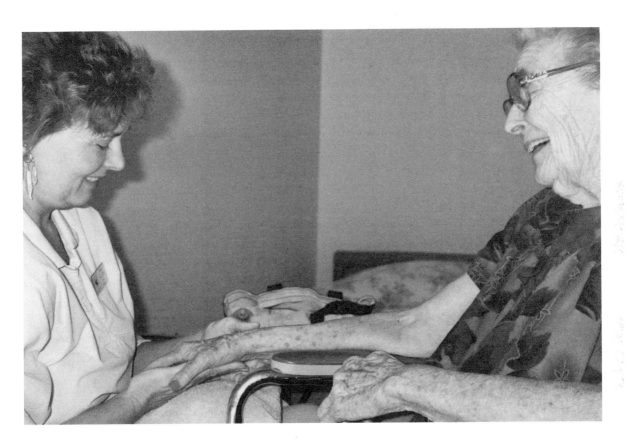

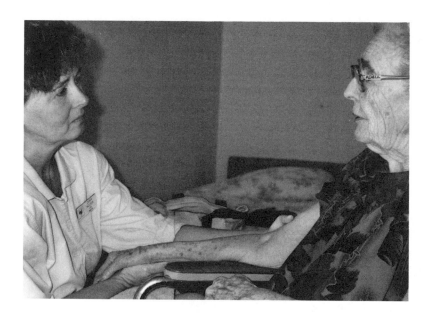

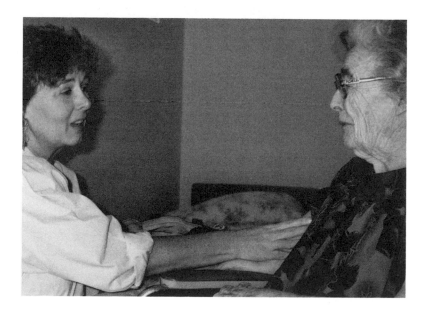

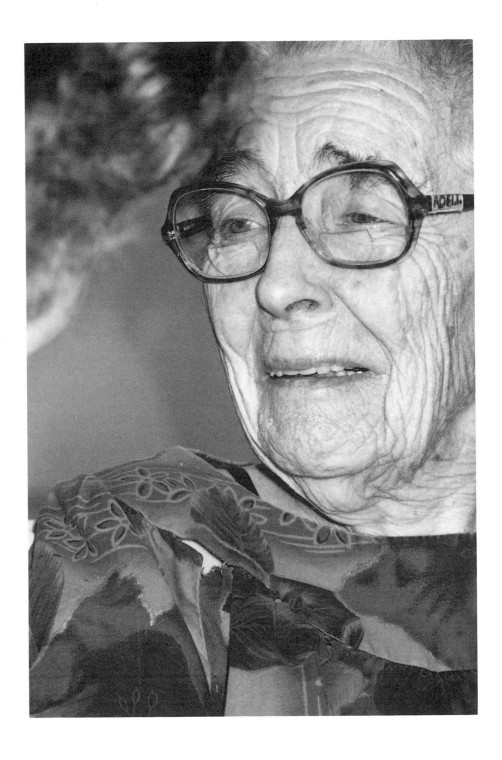

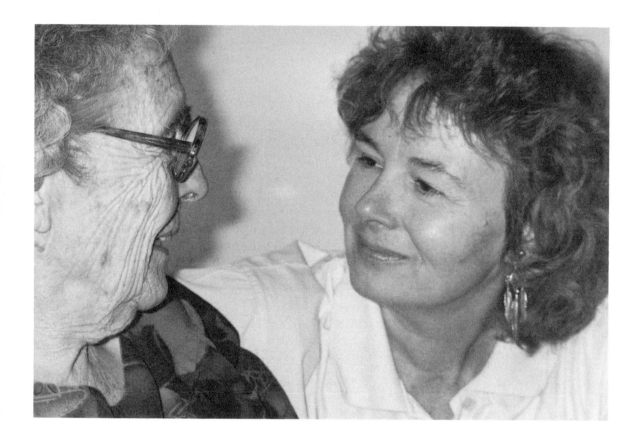

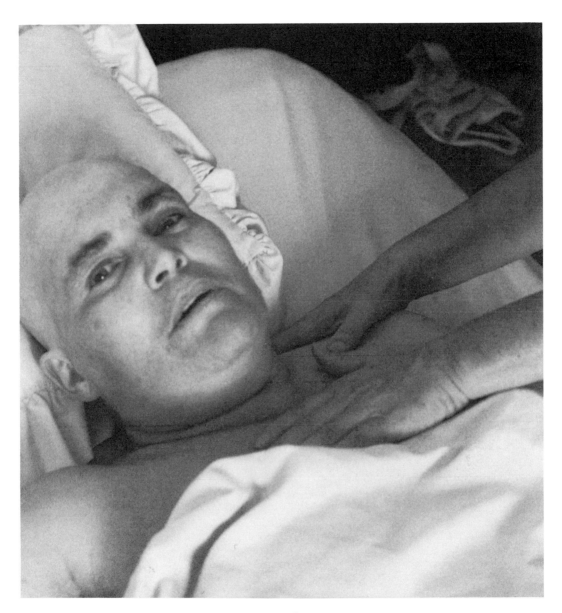

Gayle

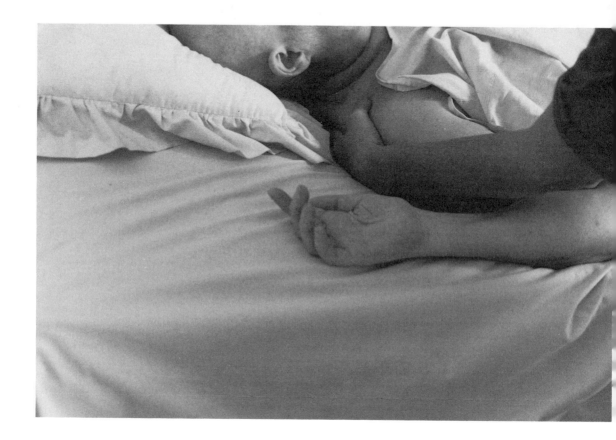

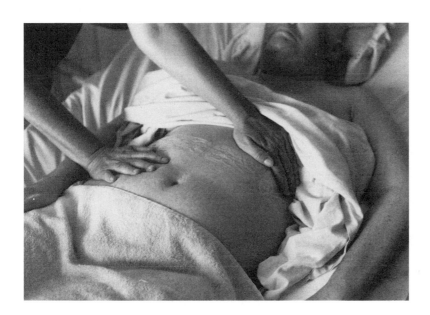

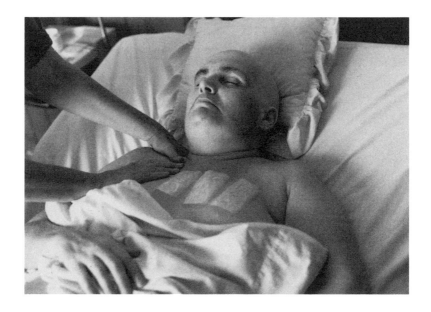

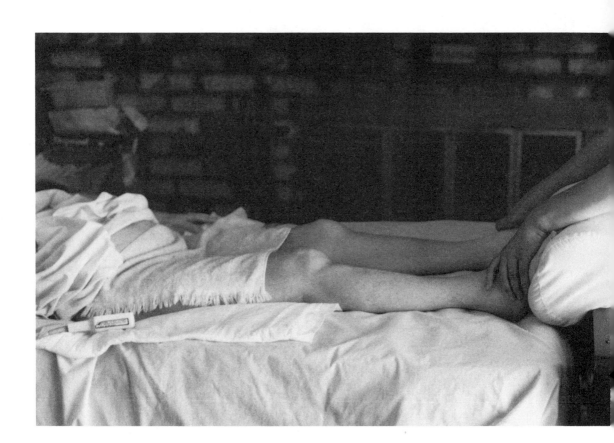

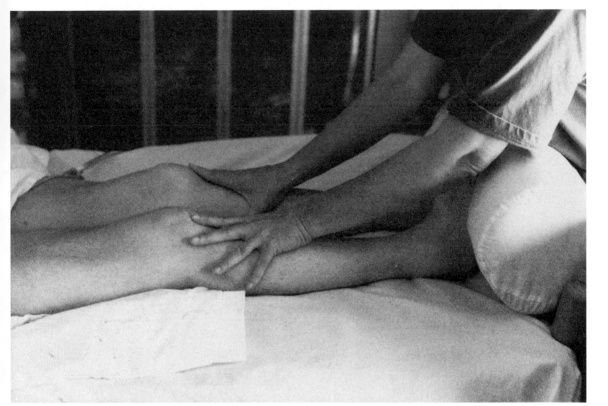

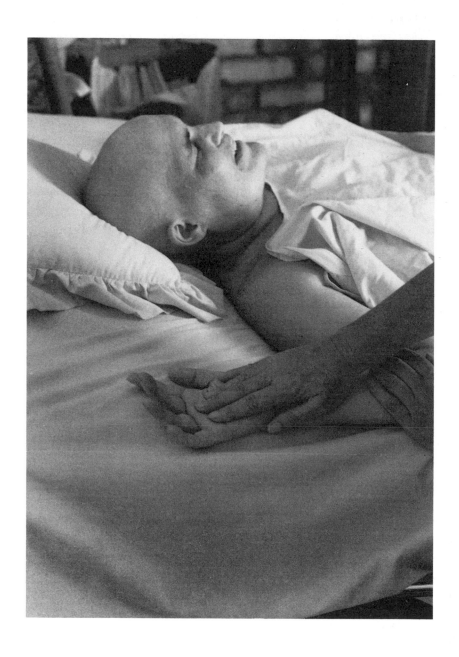

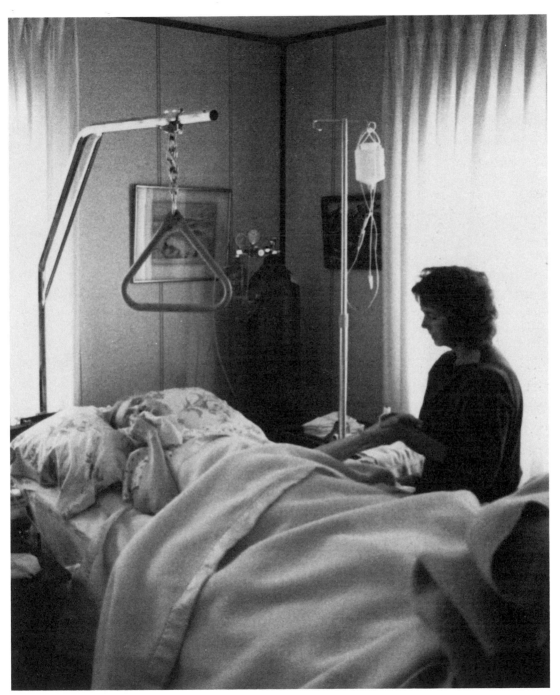

Bob

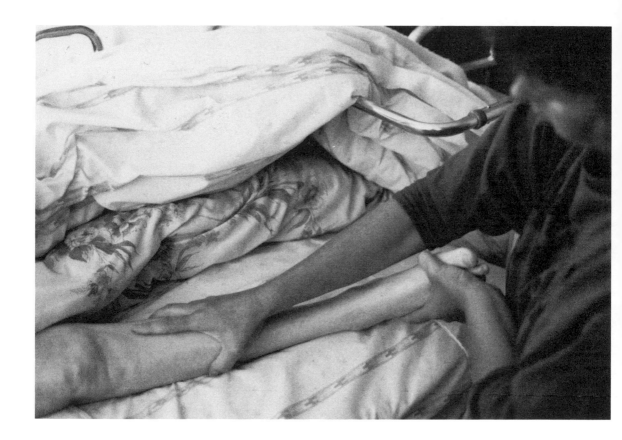

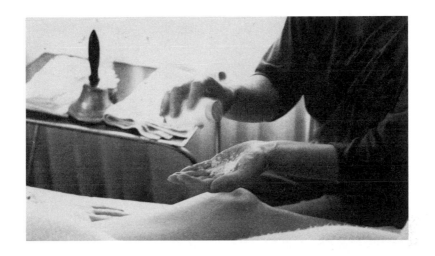

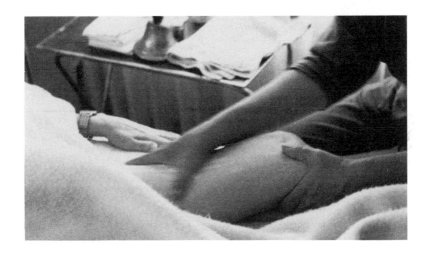

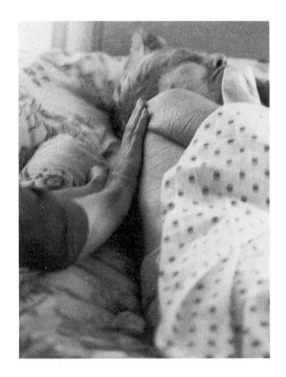

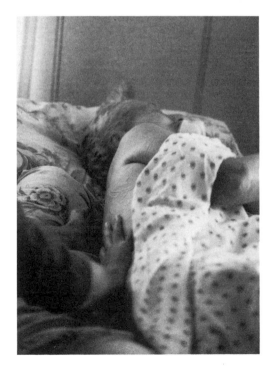

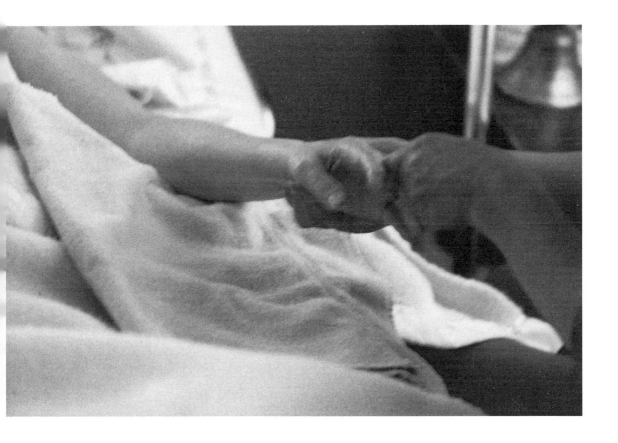

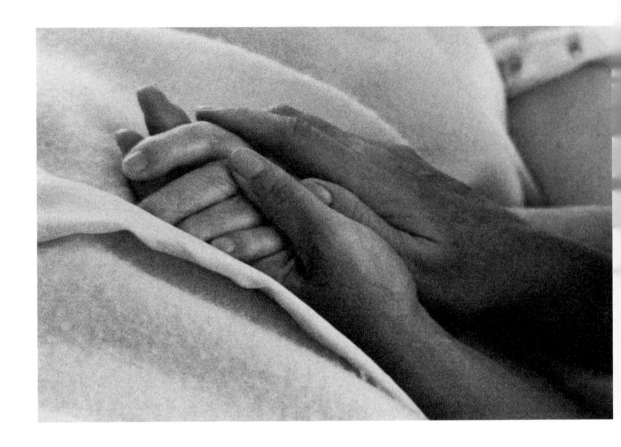

Signs of Approaching Death and Appropriate Response

These are some of the conditions or states you may observe in a person who is within a few days, hours, or minutes of death. They may not all occur. Possibly none of them will occur.

1. Body extremities become cool to the touch and may turn slightly bluish in color as blood circulation slows down. Person may complain of feeling cold.

    Use any Compassionate Touch techniques you feel are appropriate or that the person requests. Work on top of covers or reach underneath to administer massage if necessary to keep the person warm.

2. There may be an increase in time spent sleeping and some difficulty in arousal from sleep due to changing body metabolism.

    Assume that the individual can still hear everything that is being said and still experience pain. Use appropriate Compassionate Touch techniques. Sit quietly with the person. Practice shared breathing meditation as described in Chapter Six.

3. Disorientation and difficulty identifying people, time, or place, also due to changing body metabolism.

    Remain a calm and reassuring presence for the individual. Give physical and verbal contact. Tell the person who you are, where he or she is, and the names of others present in the room.

4. Decreased need for food and liquid intake as body naturally weakens and begins to conserve energy.

    Refrain from "pushing" the person to eat or drink. Respond to any requests that are made. Accept the way things are. Physical contact should be active but gentle.

5.   Incontinence (inability to control urine and/or bowel function). Urine may darken and amount passed may decrease as kidneys begin to shut down.

Help with hygiene as needed. Give sensitive verbal and physical reassurance and support. Remain focused, calm, and present.

6.   Restlessness, random hand movement, and hallucinations, which may be due, in part, to a decrease in oxygen circulation to the brain and changing body metabolism. Visions may be due to surrendered state or acceptance of death.

Accept whatever the person says, hears, or does. Remember that acknowledgement is not necessarily agreement. Maintain physical contact. Give verbal reassurance of your presence. Remain receptive and open to the individual.

7.   Irregular breathing pattern with 10-30 seconds of no breathing as circulation slows down and body waste products build up.

Breathe with the person. Maintain physical and eye contact if possible. Remain attentive and open to each moment as it unfolds.

8.   Saliva pools at back of throat, due to decrease in liquid intake, increasing weakness and inability to cough up or swallow normal saliva production. This condition may produce the noisy, congested, or gurgling sound sometimes called "death rattle."

Turn person gently onto side, support with pillows on back side, and put something under the cheek to catch secretions. Or, put a pillow under the person's head to elevate it slightly. A cool mist humidifier in the room may be helpful. Stay present and in contact with the individual.

Physical Changes in Death and Following

1. Signs that **death** has occurred include:
    Cessation of breath
    No movement
    No detectable heartbeat or pulse
    No response to verbal or physical contact
    Eyelids slightly open and eyes fixed on one spot
    Relaxed jaw leaving mouth slightly open
    Complete loss of bladder and/or bowel control

2. **Rigor mortis** (muscular rigidity) begins two to four hours after death. This contraction of muscle fibers that immobilizes the joints begins first in involuntary muscles, heart, CI tract, bladder, and arteries. It proceeds to the voluntary muscles of the head and neck and then to the trunk and lower extremities. Rigor mortis proceeds until full intensity about 48 hours after death.

3. **Algor mortis**, or cooling of the body. This is the second noticeable change after death. After circulation closes down, bodily fluids stop their movement and begin to settle. Internal body temperature begins to fall at approximately one degree per hour. Body temperature continues to drop until it approximates room temperature, which is why the skin feels cold to the touch.

4. **Decomposition.** The third major change that occurs after circulation in the body ceases is decomposition, which manifests as a softening of the tissues and discoloration making the skin appear mottled or bruised or both.

Recommended Reading

Published books devoted entirely to the subject of therapeutic massage for the elderly and the ill, or of using attentive touch with the dying do not exist to my knowledge. This particular form of comfort care is often ignored or given very short shrift in books on geriatric or long-term care. A few articles can be found on this subject but such writing is not in abundance nor is it easily accessible. This Appendix contains a partial list of books and other materials that I have used and found helpful in my own practice of therapeutic massage, in teaching, or in my personal growth as it relates to the development of Compassionate Touch.

Books Relating to Therapeutic Massage and Touch

DeLong Miller, Roberta. *Psychic Massage*. New York: Harper and Row, 1975.

Ms. Miller states that the primary purpose of her book is to inform rather than instruct—to present possibilities and potentialities—which she does very well. Simple exercises are presented that can be used to deepen one's awareness and increase one's ability to focus attention and energy while administering touch therapy and massage.

Downing, George. *The Massage Book*. Illustrated by Anne Kent Rush. New York: Random House, 1972.

One of the first, and still the best, books published on the art and practice of massage. It does not deal specifically with the subject of massaging the elderly or the ill but it is an excellent introduction to the general practice of massage as a tool for stress reduction and relaxation.

Krieger, Dolores, Ph.D., R.N. *The Therapeutic Touch: How to Use Your Hands To Help or To Heal*. Englewood Cliffs, NJ: Prentice-Hall, 1979.

Ms. Krieger, a Professor of Nursing at New York University, believes that we all have the potential of directing human energy through our hands to help or heal both ourselves and others. Her book contains a number of "self-knowledge tests" that are useful as centering practices and in learning how to detect and direct energy. Included are numerous case histories and examples of the use of Therapeutic Touch as the author defines it.

Montagu, Ashley. *Touching: The Human Significance of the Skin.* New York: Harper and Row, 1971, 1978, 1986.

This classic is a unique, well-documented and fascinating book that examines the importance of tactile interaction on human development, discusses the relationship of the skin and touching to physical and mental health, and has a thought-provoking chapter on the importance of touch for older people.

Thomas, Sara. *Massage for Common Ailments.* New York: Simon and Schuster Inc., 1988.

A well thought out and well organized book, which gives clear and instructive guidance on how to use massage to promote better health and to relieve specific problems in each area of the body. The beautiful photographs and illustrative drawings add to the clarity of the text.

Aging and Age-Related Conditions/Care

Ahn, Jung M.D. and Gary Ferguson. *Recovering from a Stroke: A Doctor's Guide for Patients and Their Loved Ones.* New York: Harper Paperbacks, 1992.

This easy-to-read book explains what a stroke is, defines medical terms in "layman's language," and separates myth from fact in terms of recovery possibilities for stroke survivors. It contains practical suggestions for physical and psychological support for working with those who have suffered a stroke and includes personal narratives from stroke survivors regarding what helps them and what does not.

Billig, Nathan, M.D. *To Be Old and Sad: Understanding Depression in the Elderly.* Lexington, MA: D.C. Heath and Co., 1987.

A useful, informative book for anyone who works with the elderly. Provides insight into why depression is so prevalent in the elderly, the signs and symptoms of depression, and how to relate to someone who is depressed. Explains what treatments are frequently used to treat this condition.

Deane, Barbara. *Caring for Your Aging Parents.* Colorado Springs: NavPress, 1989.

A chapter in this book "Coping with the Heath Problems of the Aging" is particularly helpful to those working with the elderly and/or the ill in that it describes diseases that are common in later life stages, giving symptoms, common treatments, and possible side effects of some of those treatments.

Gach, Michael Reed. *Arthritis Relief at Your Fingertips*. New York: Warner Books, 1989.

This book is a gold mine for the 35 million Americans suffering from arthritis and rheumatism and for anyone who works with the elderly. The self-help techniques outlined in this book provide relief to the victims of these crippling diseases. The clear photos and line drawings that accompany the text make it easy to learn and use the techniques, which can be taught or incorporated into therapeutic massage sessions. Cassette tapes with guidance for daily practice are also available.

Kayser-Jones, Jeanie Schmit. *Old, Alone, and Neglected: Care of the Aged in the United States and Scotland*. Berkeley: University of California Press, 1981 with 1990 Epilogues.

Written by a Professor of Medical Anthropology and Gerontological Nursing at the University of California, SF, this book is useful reading for anyone interested in working in a nursing home or extended care environment. The book is an eye-opener for those unfamiliar with the dynamics of institutional life. It provides unique insight into how and why problems such as infantilization, depersonalization, dehumanization, and victimization of residents occur within long-term care facilities.

Miller, Carol A. *Nursing Care of Older Adults: Theory and Practice*. Glenview, IL: Scott, Foresman/Little, Brown High Education, 1990.

Written by a professor of Gerontological Nursing as a comprehensive text for students, this book provides a wealth of information on older adulthood and age-related changes on all levels. Though not quickly digestible, the book is readable and informative. Much of it is useful for anyone seriously interested in working with the elderly.

Miesler, Dietrich W. *Geriatric Massage Techniques*. Guerneville, CA: Day-Break Productions, 1990.

A spiral-bound training manual for bodyworkers that is part of a series of very helpful teaching materials written by the man who founded the Day-Break Geriatric Massage Project. His emphasis is on improving the geriatric client's state of health through specific anatomy-based massage techniques. This book contains practical as well as theoretical information and is an excellent resource.

Thompson, M. Keith, M.D. *Caring for an Elderly Relative: A Guide to Home Care.* Englewood Cliffs, NJ: Prentice-Hall, 1986.

This practical and informative book contains many helpful hints about caring for, and relating to, older people. It details some of the specific issues and challenges inherent in aging on both the physical and mental levels.

Death and Dying

Callanan, Maggie and Patricia Kelly. *FINAL GIFTS.* New York: Bantam Books, 1992.

A compassionate, insightful, illuminating, and practical book that will be helpful and encouraging to anyone working with the dying and is a real treasure for caregivers. Written by two Hospice nurses, the book helps the reader understand the special needs of the dying, how to communicate with those nearing death, and how to remain open to receiving the unique gifts those individuals have to offer.

Hamilton, Michael and Helen Reid, eds. *The Hospice Handbook: A New Way to Care For the Dying.* Grand Rapids, MI: William B. Eerdmans Publishing, 1980.

A good resource book for anyone interested in working with Hospice or with the dying in general. Gives a history of the Hospice concept and goals. The personal essays in Part I are particularly useful in providing insight into the needs of the seriously ill.

Kubler-Ross, Elisabeth. *AIDS.* New York: Macmillan Publishing Company, 1987.

Elisabeth Kubler-Ross has spent most of her life working with seriously ill people of all ages and familiarizing others with the needs, concerns, and fears of individuals facing the end of life. This unique book challenges, inspires, and educates the reader in regard to every aspect of what may be the world's most serious health crisis—the AIDS epidemic.

Kubler-Ross, Elisabeth, photographs by Mal Warshaw. *To Live Until We Say Good-bye.* Englewood Cliffs, NJ: Prentice-Hall, 1978.

A profoundly moving and compassionate work that contains thought-provoking text along with heart-opening visual images of individuals of different ages who, along with their loved ones, volunteers, and friends, share their process in facing life-threatening illness and death. This book is intimate, positive, and powerfully eloquent.

Levine, Stephen. *Healing into Life and Death*. Garden City, NY: Anchor Press/ Doubleday, 1987.

Thought-provoking and investigative into the nature of what true healing is, this compassionate guide offers techniques for working with pain and grief and for developing merciful awareness in regard to ourselves as well as in relationship to others.

Levine, Stephen. *Meetings at the Edge: Dialogues with the Grieving and the Dying, the Healing and the Healed*. Garden City, NY: Anchor Press/ Doubleday 1984.

For a period of about three years, Stephen and his wife offered a free consultation phone for the "terminally ill and those working closely with a death." This book is a sharing of a number of those conversations. The dialogues are intimate, moving, and enlightening.

Levine, Stephen. *Who Dies? An Investigation of Conscious Living and Conscious Dying*. Garden City, NY: Anchor Press/Doubleday, 1982.

This book is just what the title says it is. Read with an open mind and heart, it might change one's perspective about living and about dying significantly. Essential, though not "easy," reading for any serious student of life/death.

Grief and Bereavement

Donnelley, Nina Herrmann. *I Never Know What To Say: How to Help Your Family and Friends Cope with Tragedy*. New York: Ballentine Books, 1987.

A book that is helpful in its personal insights about facing death, the various aspects of mourning a loss, and what to say to others who are grieving. It contains a short section on the importance of touching those who are ill and/or close to death.

Elaine Childs-Gowell.*Good Grief Rituals*. Barrytown, NY: Station Hill Press, NY, 1992.

A gentle book that contains simple exercises and tools for dealing with loss of any kind. A treasure box of tools for the healing and integration process!

Tatelbaum, Judy. *The Courage to Grieve: Creative Living, Recovery, & Growth Through Grief*. New York: Harper and Row, 1980.

A truly helpful book, well written with compassion and sensitivity, on all aspects of grief and grief resolution. A valuable aid to anyone who works with the aged, the seriously ill, and the grieving.

Caregiver Support

Ronch, Judah L. *Alzheimer's Disease: A Practical Guide for Families and Other Caregivers.* New York: Continuum, 1991.

A sensitive, well-written, and informative book on this specific form of dementia and its impact on individuals and their families. Gives practical and wise advice for accepting and respecting the person who is suffering from this disease while dealing with the challenges of living with, or caring for, such a person.

Baulch, Evelyn M. *Extended Health Care at Home.* Berkeley, CA: Celestial Arts, 1988.

As the cover notes, this book is a complete and practical guide for home caregivers. It covers every aspect of home care and includes chapters on caring for the elderly, for children, for the handicapped, for those with AIDS, for the seriously ill and the dying. The author describes the physical and emotional drain such care entails as well as the joy and satisfaction it can bring. An excellent resource and reference book.

Little, Deborah Whiting. *Home Care for the Dying.* Garden City, NY: Doubleday, 1985.

Certain sections of this book give practical guidance and useful information for anyone who might be involved in serving or helping care for someone who is ill and/or elderly in a home setting. This book also addresses the issue of stress faced by family members caring for a loved one who is facing death.

Mace, Nancy L. and Peter V. Rabins. *The 36-Hour Day*, revised edition. Baltimore, MD: Johns Hopkins University Press, 1991.

This book contains a wealth of clear information designed to help the reader understand the characteristics of dementing ilnesses and how to relate to those who exhibit such characteristics. In addition to sharing the latest research available on all forms of dementia, it gives invaluable practical advice and guidance. I have heard more than one caregiver say that *"THE 36-HOUR DAY* saved my life."

Self-Care

Benson, Herbert. *The Relaxation Response.* New York: Wm. Morrow, 1975.

This book helps the reader in identifying and evaluating personal stress. It includes a scientific study of medication and its effects on the physical body, and it outlines the author's theory that the body will relax if changes are first made in one's mental state. Practical suggestions and exercises for evoking the relaxation response are given.

Gach, Michael Reed. *Accupressure's Potent Points: A Guide to Self-Care for Common Ailments.* New York: Bantam, 1990.

One of the best self-help books I know of for anyone striving for a healthy and balanced life. This book makes the ancient healing art of finger pressure accessible to modern wo/man. The author reveals simple, learnable techniques that enable the reader to relieve more than forty common ailments and symptoms using the power and sensitivity of his or her own hands. Photographs of real people practicing the techniques outlined in the text, as well as easy-to-read line drawings, enhance this book.

Weil, Andrew, M.D. *Natural Health, Natural Medicine: A Comprehensive Manual for Wellness and Self-Care.* Boston, MA: Houghton Mifflin Co., 1990.

Working within the medical profession and advocating natural medicine and self-care as a legitimate alternative to conventional medical treatment, Dr. Weil has compiled a great deal of information into a practical, clear, readable, and highly useful health guide. An invaluable resource for health maintenance, the book outlines specific preventive measures to take in order to avoid debilitating diseases and protect the immune system.

Other Helpful Books

Sohnen-Moe, Cherie. *Business Mastery.* Tuscon, AZ: Sohnen-Moe Associates, 1991.

This planning guide for creating a fulfilling, successful business is designed especially for healing arts professionals. The author's stated purpose in writing the book is to "assist you in having your business be an expression of creativity, joy, empowerment, balance, and profitability." A valuable resource for anyone who wants to achieve success in the business world while staying true to the highest principles of healing and service to others.

Levine, Stephen. *Guided Meditations, Explorations and Healings.* Garden City, NY: Anchor Books/Doubleday, 1991.

Guided meditations, mindfulness practices, and processes for self-awareness that may be used for personal exploration and relaxation, or in working with others. Any of the meditations can be adapted to your own style and then read aloud or recorded on tape to give as gifts.

Carlson, Richard and Benjamin Shield, editors. *Healers on Healing.* Los Angeles, CA: Jeremy P. Tarcher, 1989.

An anthology of essays written by nearly forty different well-known, non-traditional healers who explore the nature of healing from various viewpoints. Some topics addressed include: love as a healing force, the effects of healing relationships, the power of the healer within, healing and death, and how healing takes place.

Ram Dass and Paul Gorman. *HOW CAN I HELP? Stories and Reflections on Service.* New York: Alfred A. Knopf, 1986.

A wise and wonderful book that offers practical guidance as well as inspiration, through deeply moving personal stories of caring and compassion. Thoughtful and useful reading for anyone who is interested in "helping" others.

Additional Resources

National Alzheimer's Association, 70 E. Lake, Suite 600, Chicago, IL, 60601. Telephone 1-800-621-0379.

National Hospice Organization, 1901 N. Moore Drive, Suite 901, Arlington, VA 22209. Telephone 703-684-7722.

National Institute on Aging, National Institutes of Health, 7550 Wisconsin Avenue, Room 618, Bethesda, MD 20892. Telephone 301-496-5345.

Service Through Touch, 41 Carl Street #C; San Francisco, California 94117

Founded by Irene Smith in 1982 as a volunteer program offering massage to AIDS patients, Service Through Touch is now a non-profit corporation dedicated to integrating touch and massage into health care for the seriously ill. Service Through Touch provides written, audio, and visual materials on massaging people with H.I.V. Disease.

About the Author

   Dawn Nelson has been a professional practitioner and teacher of therapeutic massage as a healing art since 1978. Once a professional actress, Dawn is also an experienced group facilitator, communications counselor, and meditation teacher. In 1991, after completing an innovative academic Certification in Working With the Dying as part of a graduate program in counseling psychology, Dawn founded Compassionate Touch For Those in Later Life Stages, an outreach service offering therapeutic massage and attentive touch to the elderly and the ill in health care, home, and hospice settings. Dawn offers Compassionate Touch training to massage therapists, health care professionals, and volunteer caregivers nationwide. The mother of three, Dawn lives with her husband and youngest child in Walnut Creek, California.

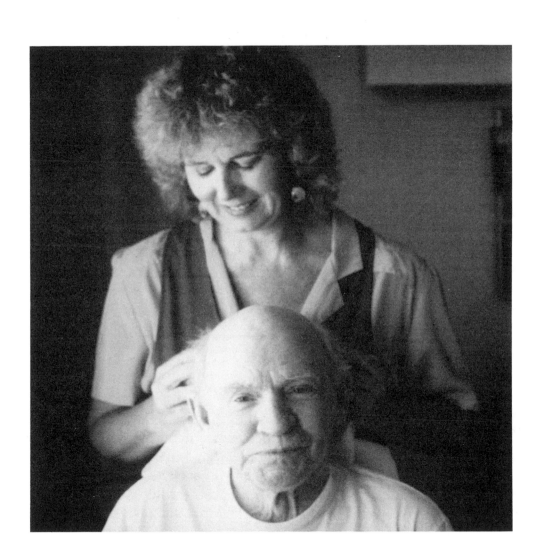

If you have any questions or comments about this book, or about Compassionate Touch training programs, videos or services, please contact:

Compassionate Touch
20 Swan Court
Walnut Creek, California 94596
Phone: (510) 935-3906

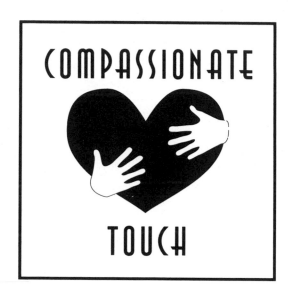

Compassionate Touch: Benefits and Effects in Long Term Care

This high quality, color video is an illuminating guide for health care professionals and facility administrators as well as for massage therapists and bodyworkers
interested in enhancing quality of life for the elderly and the ill. Elucidates both
the physical and psycho-social benefits of one-on-one attention in the form of
therapeutic touch and massage for residents of care facilities, emphasizing the
importance of the relationship between the therapist and resident. Details the
successful implementation of the Compassionate Touch program in an extended care hospital, including promotion, billing and evaluation procedures.
Innerlight Productions, 23 minutes VHS $39.95. Videos are available from Station Hill
Press, Station Hill Rd., Barrytown, New York, 12507, (914) 758-5840.

Discount Schedule:

1-7 copies	8-15 copies	16-25 copies	25 or more copies
$39.95 per copy	$31.96 (20% disc.)	$27.96 (30% disc.)	$23.97 (40% disc.)

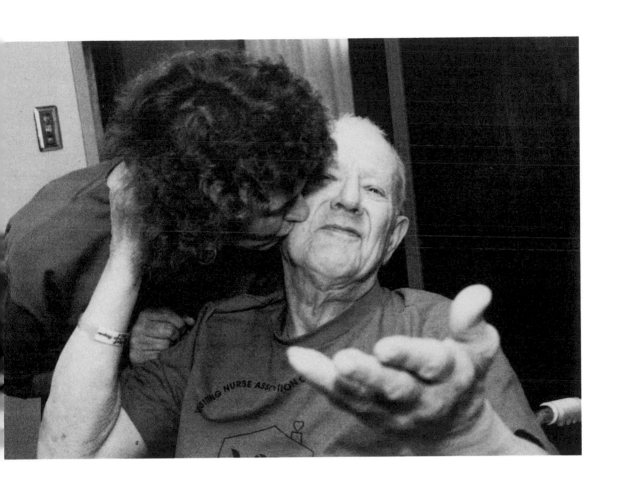

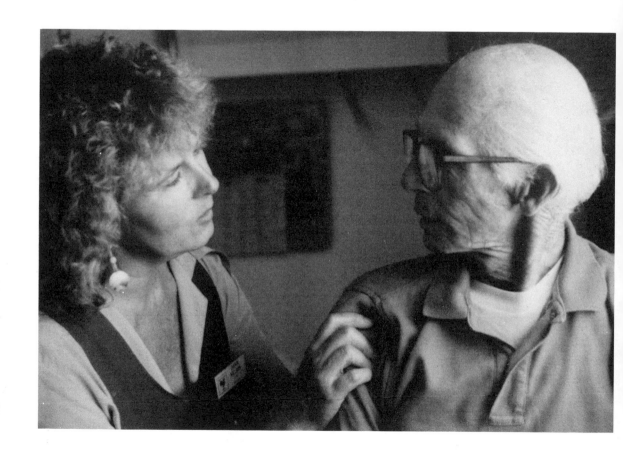

May we all live in mercy and care for each other and for ourselves. May we all come to treasure ourselves and each other. And may we all come to treasure each other in ourselves.

Stephen Levine

Index

National Institute on Aging 165
nervous tension 5
nurture 13-14

oils — see lotion
on-site massage therapy 105, 106
Orthobionomy 43
oxygen 6, 7, 14, 15, 32, 82, 89, 156

pain xi, xiii 5, 6; 8, 9, 17, 21, 25, 30,
31, 32, 33, 85, 86, 102, 103,
104, 111, 112, 113, 116
positive and negative responses, 87
powder 8, 37
preconceived ideas 25, 81
pressure 7, 15, 27, 45, 46, 51, 57 62,
67, 84, 89
pressure massage 46, 47, 48, 49, 52
processing grief 113
protecting yourself 83, 84
protection 84, 92, 93
psoriasis 8
psychic touch 45, 66
psycho-social benefits 12, 18-21

Rabins, Peter V. 163
Ram Dass 35
range of motion 13, 45, 68, 69
Reid Helen 161
reflective reedback 70, 87
relaxation 5, 6, 8, 17, 39, 71, 73, 87,
88, 105, 112, 113, 164
renewed vitality 14
responsiveness 5, 6, 9, 10, 14, 15, 17,
19, 20, 45, 70
rigor mortis 157
rhomboid muscles 46
Ronch, Judah L. 163
Rosen Work 43

Schmit Kayser-Jones 79
self, sense of 26-27
self-care 111, 164
self-esteem 14, 20, 95
sense memory 17-18, 73
sensitive massage 45-46
Service Through Touch 179
sexual energy 91

shared breathing 74-75
Shield, Benjamin 165
shifting 7, 45, 67, 68
skin 7, 8, 9, 18, 36, 37, 38, 46, 51,
62, 63, 67, 73, 80, 83, 92, 93,
95, 106
  contagious problems 83-84
  lotion applied to 35-36, 46
  prevention of problems 7-8
  rashes 84
  weeping lesions 84
Smith, Irene 23, 93, 165
social interaction 11, 18
Sohnen-Mae, Cherie 164
squeezing 46, 50, 57
stress xi, 5, 6, 8, 9, 10, 20, 71, 72,
103, 104, 105, 111, 112, 163
stretching 45, 67, 80, 88
stroke 10, 16, 55, 68, 87, 96
stroking 13, 15, 18, 45, 46, 51, 52, 55,
56, 58, 67, 83, 106
subconscious 25
support for at home caregivers 103
Swanson, Donna 12

Tatelbaum, Judy 162
tension 5, 6, 8, 9, 10, 13, 72, 80
Thomas, Sara 159
Thompson, M. Keith, M.D. 160
thrombophlebitis 83
thrombosis 83
Tiger Balm 38
touch deprivation 12
touch therapy 7,
touching 5, 7, 8, 16, 17, 18, 19, 39,
40, 43, 45, 46, 62, 63, 66,
72, 74, 79, 80, 82, 83, 84, 93,
97, 165
Trager Approach 43

vitality, renewed 14-15
visions 44, 77
visualization 71, 72, 73
  see also guided fantasy
  see also creative visualization

weight loss 94
Weil, Andrew, M.D. 164

Related Titles from Station Hill Press

How to Forgive When You Don't Know How
JACQUI BISHOP & MARY GRUNTE

In this groundbreaking look at the psychology of forgiveness, the authors show how resentment — toward other people, towards one's self, even toward God — can consume precious emotional energy and seriously impair both self-esteem and the ability to experience joy. Drawing on the healing techniques used so successfully in *How to Love Yourself When You Don't Know How*, they offer a short program for accelerating the process of forgiveness, including visualization, emotional discharge, searching back, and prayer. Enlivened with classic quotations on the nature of forgiveness, this revolutionary book explodes long-standing myths — including the notion that forgiveness involves self-denial, making up, confessing, or turning the other cheek. Its easy-to-use format puts it on the shelf with *Good Grief Rituals*.

$8.95 paper, ISBN 0-88268-142-7

Movement as a Way to Agelessness
A Guide to Trager Mentastics
MILTON TRAGER, M.D., WITH CATHY GUADAGNO, PH.D.

Trager Mentastics helped people of all ages achieve greater flexibility, coordination, and balance, as well as the lightness of being its author calls "agelessness." Now this expanded edition, with all-new photos and additional movements, re-introduces this profoundly simple system of dancelike movements for the body and mind to all those looking not just to extend life but to reduce aging itself. The method is also known to help victims of polio, muscular dystrophy, respiratory problems, MS, lower back pain, and chronic aches and pains.

$15.95 paper, ISBN 0-88268-167-2

Related Titles from Station Hill Press

Emotional First Aid
A Crisis Handbook
SEAN HALDANE, M.D.

Emotional First Aid is the first book to address immediate emotional crisis as distinct from a person's general state of mental health. It deals with grief, anger, fear, joy, and also the complex feelings of parent/child conflicts — emotions that can lead to further withdrawal, illness, or even violence. Clear and extraordinarily well written, this is the first book to draw on Reichian character analysis to explain how differences in individuals and in specific emotions call for different responses, if one is to be supportive and not invasive. Emotional first aid may precede or prevent therapy in the same way that physical first aid can precede or prevent extended medical treatment.

$9.95 paper, ISBN 0-88268-071-4

Osteoarthritis
A Step-by-Step Success Story to Show Others They Can Help Themselves
FRED L. SAVAGE

In 1985 Fred Savage was painfully crippled with osteoarthritis; the simplest tasks — driving a car, walking up a flight of stairs — became nearly impossible. His own remarkable return to a pain-free life forms the basis of this clearly written and exceedingly useful book. Though osteoarthritis remains incurable, the author asserts that it is eminently manageable, through a combination of exercise, walking, Trager bodywork and Mentastics, and relaxation. He introduces a range of useful products, from special shoes to orthopedic supports, and describes how simple changes in everyday life, including increased rest periods, better ways of walking and sitting, and a healthier diet, can successfully keep osteoarthritis under control. Drawn from personal experience, this sensible and comprehensible book will be welcomed by the more than 20 million people who suffer from osteoarthritis.

$11.95 paper, ISBN 0-88268-086-2.

Related Titles from Station Hill Press

Job's Body
A Handbook for Bodywork
DEANE JUHAN
Foreword by Ken Dychtwald

One of the hallmarks of the renaissance of bodywork in America, *Job's Body* is now considered the preeminent text on its subject. The book demonstrates the power of bodywork to alter the course of a wide range of ailments and provides the most authoritative account to date of how the body responds to touch. Writing in a style accessible to lay and professional readers alike, Deane Juhan offers a synthesis of scientific, historical, and experiential data to support the claims of a variety of techniques, among them Rolfing, Feldenkreis, Trager, and Alexander methods, shiatsu, re-birthing, acupressure, zero-balancing, bioenergetics, trigger-point therapy, and massage. Especially timely are the author's suggestions on how skilled manipulation can be incorporated into traditional methods of health care.

$24.95 paper, ISBN 0-88268-134-6, $49.95 cloth, ISBN 0-88268-047-1

Related Titles from Station Hill Press

Good Grief Rituals
Tools for Healing
ELAINE CHILDS-GOWELL

As a psychotherapist with over twenty year's experience, the author realized that the emotion of grief was not limited to bereavement but was in fact experienced in an extraordinary range of circumstances, from natural disasters to the end of a love affair. In this sane, comforting, and deeply thoughtful book, she offers the reader a series of simple grief rituals, among them the venting of feelings, letter writing, affirmations, exercises to act out negative emotions as well as forgiveness, fantasies, meditations, and more. Adult chidren of alcoholics and dysfunctional families, victims of incest and assault, and those who've lost a pet, wrecked a car, or suffered any kind of loss will find that these "good grief rituals" move them through loss to forgiveness and, ultimately, to gratitude and a new sense of life.

$8.95p, ISBN 0-88268-118-4; 112 pages, 6 x 6 ½.